FAQs on Dementia

FAQs on Dementia

TOM RUSS AND
MICHAEL HUDDLESTON

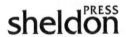

First published in Great Britain by Sheldon Press in 2023
An imprint of John Murray Press
A division of Hodder & Stoughton Ltd,
An Hachette UK company

3

This book is for information or educational purposes only and is not
intended to act as a substitute for medical advice or treatment. Any
person with a condition requiring medical attention should consult a
qualified medical practitioner or suitable therapist.

A CIP catalogue record for this title is available from the British Library

Trade Paperback ISBN 9781399802550
eBook ISBN 9781399802567

Typeset by KnowledgeWorks Global Ltd.

Printed and bound in Great Britain by Clays Ltd, Elcograf S.p.A.

John Murray Press policy is to use papers that are natural, renewable and
recyclable products and made from wood grown in sustainable forests.
The logging and manufacturing processes are expected to conform to the
environmental regulations of the country of origin.

John Murray Press
Carmelite House
50 Victoria Embankment
London EC4Y 0DZ

www.sheldonpress.co.uk

For John, who suggested I write a book – TR

For the people living with dementia and carers
I spend time with, whose experiences transcend
anything a book could possibly capture – MH

Contents

About the authors

Dr Tom Russ PhD FRCPsych is a consultant psychiatrist in NHS Lothian and an honorary clinical reader at the University of Edinburgh. He has worked in the NHS since 2004 from Caithness in the north of Scotland to West Sussex on the south coast of England and several places in between. His PhD focused on risk factors for dementia, particularly whether where you live and environmental risk factors are important. He is Director of the Alzheimer Scotland Dementia Research Centre at the University of Edinburgh and Clinical Research Champion of the NHS Research Scotland (NRS) Neuroprogressive and Dementia Network.

Michael Huddleston is Alzheimer Scotland's Dementia Advisor for Mid and East Lothian. He provides advice and information for people living with dementia and their families, and works closely with local Health and Social Care Partnerships to influence and shape dementia and carer-specific strategies and to accommodate the needs and views of people with lived experience.

Foreword

The Scottish Dementia Working Group and the National Dementia Carers Action Network

The Scottish Dementia Working Group (SDWG) and National Dementia Carers Action Network (NDCAN) are national member-led groups, for people living with a diagnosis of dementia and carers of people with dementia. As active voice groups, our members are committed to enabling and promoting the diverse voices of people with dementia and carers to campaign for, promote and uphold rights and drive change. Our priorities include raising awareness, improving rights, and tackling the stigma of dementia.

Alongside what unites us, it is important to remember that no two people impacted by dementia are the same. We are all different, with different needs and different interests. Some of us like to sing or play music, others enjoy keeping active or being creative. There are those who want to continue working or learning, whilst maintaining social connections with friends and family is a priority for others.

Just as our interests are different, so too are our experiences of dementia. Every person's dementia journey is different, from the pathway to diagnosis, to living well with dementia. And, from how we can keep doing the things we enjoy, to managing the symptoms of dementia and the support we might need.

Working together has shown us that there's no one-size-fits-all answer to dementia, but there are common questions that arise and helpful advice and useful information that can be shared. This book sets out to do just that and provides insight on everything from what dementia is and how it is diagnosed, to the symptoms and stages of dementia, how to live well with dementia and how to support someone living with dementia.

Alongside answers to the many questions that people living with dementia and their carers have, you'll find helpful suggestions and strategies to assist both the person living with dementia and those who support them to adapt to and cope with changes in memory and behaviour. There's also an important chapter for carers with advice and information on self-care.

In producing this book Tom and Michael have brought together their wealth of knowledge and experience to create an excellent and long overdue resource for anyone affected by dementia, and we hope you will find it to be an effective guide as you navigate your own dementia journey.

Preface

Whether you are worried about your memory, have been diagnosed with dementia, or are concerned on behalf of a friend or relative, we hope you find the answers to your questions in this book. No one should have to go through dementia alone, and we hope you have support around you and can find extra help as you need it.

One difficulty in writing a book like this is not knowing who is reading. We have tried to be consistent, but there are times when we address the person with dementia and others where the information is aimed at their relative or carer (not only are there text boxes addressed to carers throughout but Chapters 18 and 19 are addressed exclusively to them). Similarly, it is easier to see if the information is pitched at the correct level or is too convoluted in conversation than on the page. We have attempted to be clear while also including some detail for those who want to know more. We have done our best to achieve a reasonable balance.

We used Twitter and our local contacts to source the questions people with dementia and their families thought were important. Hopefully, this approach means that the book will be helpful to many people. We are very grateful to friends and colleagues who posed questions or have read all or some of this book in manuscript form. In particular, we would like to thank Alzheimer Scotland for permission to reproduce Figures 7.1 and 15.1, Rosie Ashworth, Willy Gilder, Fiona Hartley, Stuart Hay, Emma Law, Donncha Mullin, David Ross, Lucy Stirland, Danielle Wilson, and all the Partners in Research who read the manuscript. Their comments have greatly enriched this book. The responsibility for any remaining mistakes or infelicities of language is, of course, ours.

Finally, we are grateful to our families for their love and support while we were typing, and always.

Tom Russ and Michael Huddleston
Autumn 2022

1

What is dementia?

Doesn't everyone's memory get worse as they get older?

Some human faculties worsen as part of 'normal' ageing. The ability that most commonly deteriorates is reaction time. A slower reaction time can make it harder to process information quickly. It can mean you take longer to think things through and make decisions.

Other faculties, like wisdom, often – but not always! – continue to increase into later life. Similarly, our vocabulary tends to increase and then remains stable throughout life.

Memory problems are often assumed to be one of the normal aspects of getting older. However, if you struggle to remember things, it might actually signal that something other than ageing is happening.

Do memory problems mean that I have dementia?

If you are experiencing memory problems, you should contact your doctor and arrange an assessment. However, don't jump to the conclusion that you have dementia. That is a possibility, but there are plenty of other reasons why you might be experiencing memory problems. Of approximately 1000 people referred to our memory clinic in Edinburgh each year, probably half are diagnosed with dementia. Other reasons a person's memory might worsen include side effects from medication, other health conditions, stress, depression and anxiety. You can do something about most of these conditions, either through changing medications or lifestyle. As such, it is very important to contact your doctor if you or your family are concerned about your memory.

The dementia syndrome

Medicine was previously much more straightforward, and the branch of medicine that dealt with the mind especially so. There is a bust of the famous French doctor Philippe Pinel (1745–1826) in the hospital where Tom works. Rather than the thousands of coded illnesses in the World Health Organization's latest International Classification of Diseases, Pinel recognized only four diagnoses: melancholia (which we now call depression), mania, idiocy (intellectual disability), and dementia.

The word 'dementia' comes from the Latin *demens*, meaning 'out of one's mind', but is now used to denote a syndrome (a collection of symptoms that often go together):

- a deterioration in one or more cognitive (thinking) skills, often including memory
- experience of difficulties when carrying out everyday tasks
- progressive deterioration (i.e. it keeps getting worse)
- deterioration lasting at least six months.

Is Alzheimer's the same as dementia?

Several different illnesses can cause the syndrome of dementia. The most common is Alzheimer disease, which is probably why many people think dementia and Alzheimer's are the same.

However, clinicians are often to blame for this uncertainty because of the imprecise way we use language. To be precise, we must distinguish between Alzheimer *disease* and Alzheimer *dementia* (often formerly referred to as 'dementia in Alzheimer disease'). Alzheimer disease is an illness which affects the brain. It can be detected in people's brains even when they are only in their thirties or forties.

These changes in the brain tend to get worse with age, but – importantly – not everyone who has Alzheimer disease goes on to develop Alzheimer dementia. The latter is a progressive decline in memory (and other thinking skills) and other day-to-day abilities. Simply put, Alzheimer disease affects the brain, and Alzheimer dementia affects the person.

Many people with Alzheimer disease in their brain will likely never develop any symptoms of Alzheimer dementia. Unfortunately, we cannot currently predict who will develop symptoms and end up with a diagnosis of Alzheimer dementia, and who will live to a ripe old age with no memory problems and die of something else, despite having Alzheimer disease in their brain.

Is dementia the same as Alzheimer's?

Many other illnesses also cause dementia, so no – dementia and Alzheimer dementia are not the same. Nevertheless, Alzheimer disease is the illness that most commonly results in dementia.

Vascular dementia

The second most common illness is cerebrovascular disease, or changes in the blood vessels within the brain. This same process occurs throughout the body and can also lead to angina and ischaemic heart disease. Vascular disease causes small areas of the brain either to be starved of oxygen over a long period or die. This can lead to vascular dementia (dementia resulting from cerebrovascular disease).

Vascular dementia can occur alongside one or more strokes or 'transient ischaemic attacks' (TIAs, or mini-strokes). Dementia symptoms after a large stroke are called 'post-stroke dementia'. The underlying process in the brain is the same.

Mixed dementia

Many people diagnosed with dementia have a combination of Alzheimer dementia and cerebrovascular disease. This combination is generally referred to as 'mixed dementia'.

Dementia with Lewy bodies

The next most common overall cause of dementia (but the second most common *neurodegenerative* cause at 10–15 per cent) is dementia with Lewy bodies. 'Lewy bodies' (build ups of protein in the brain) are named after Dr Frederic Lewy (1880–1950), the Jewish German doctor who first identified these features in the brain in 1910.

Frontotemporal lobar degeneration syndromes

The fourth most common cause of dementia is the frontotemporal lobar degeneration syndromes. These all predominantly affect the frontal and temporal lobes of the brain. Symptoms include changes in behaviour or language with particular difficulties with executive function (planning and sequencing).

What about less common illnesses associated with dementia?

The four common causes make up about 19 out of 20 dementia diagnoses. However, there are further causes of dementia, including progressive supranuclear palsy, Huntington disease, motor neuron disease, corticobasal degeneration, cerebral amyloid angiopathy, CADASIL (cerebral autosomal dominant arteriopathy with subcortical infarcts and leukoencephalopathy), and Creutzfeldt–Jakob disease. There isn't room to discuss these conditions in detail here, but information is available online. A good place to start is the websites of general dementia charities or those for the specific disease. (e.g. see pg148)

Does dementia run in families? What does it mean for my children if I have dementia?

Some dementias do run in families, but these tend to be the types of illness where, tragically, people develop symptoms much earlier than usual, often in their forties. They are usually associated with known genetic abnormalities, and several people in the wider family might be affected. Someone with a mutation in one of the relevant genes has a 50/50 chance of passing it on to their children.

Most people who develop dementia do so later in life (often arbitrarily defined as 65 years or older), and age is the most important risk factor. That is not to say that genetics doesn't play a role. Someone with a first-degree relative (a parent, sibling or child) who has Alzheimer dementia has a slightly increased risk of developing dementia compared to the general population. Still, many people with a close relative with dementia do not develop dementia.

Except for those rare genetic instances mentioned above, it is not inevitable that someone who has a relative with dementia will develop dementia themself.

2

When does dementia start?

Isn't dementia a disease of old age?

Traditionally, dementia has been regarded as something that happens to people in later life. In *As You Like It*, Shakespeare described the last stage of life as 'sans teeth, sans eyes, sans taste, sans everything'. While we won't argue with the Bard, it is increasingly recognized that, although the symptoms of cognitive and functional decline most commonly occur in later life, the underlying disease process begins years, if not decades, earlier. Disease – for example, Alzheimer disease – is not the same as dementia. Disease comes before dementia.

When does the risk of developing dementia start?

Rather than a disease of later life, dementia should be understood as a disease of the whole life course. In other words, your risk of developing dementia starts to accumulate before birth. Genetic factors (which you inherit from your parents) can influence your risk of developing dementia before you were even conceived, in the selection of which egg your mother released and which of your father's sperm fertilized that egg.

What happens to you in the womb is also relevant to your subsequent health. Our experience in the womb (the 'intrauterine environment') affects the risk of developing coronary heart disease later in life. A similar relationship with the brain has also been identified. A recent study showed that people who were small babies performed more poorly on cognitive tests 70 years later, other things being equal. Admittedly, there is limited evidence directly linking birth characteristics with dementia, but many scientists are beginning to make an association between smaller birth weight and higher dementia risk later in life.

Once you are born, your experiences continue to influence your later risk of dementia. Your early life experience matters.

When does Alzheimer disease begin in the brain?

The development of Alzheimer disease – and many diseases which cause dementia – is initially silent, causing no symptoms. It begins many years before any symptoms appear. Some people, despite having a substantial amount of brain disease, never develop symptoms of dementia. We do not yet know why some people's brains seem more resilient against the changes of Alzheimer disease than others, although there are several theories.

What is cognitive reserve?

Cognitive reserve is one theory – often associated with Professor Yaakov Stern of Columbia University in New York City – to explain why some people's brains are more resilient against the changes that can result in dementia. People have different numbers of brain cells – we call this 'brain reserve' – and some people's brains also try to compensate for any damage to the brain. As we know, Alzheimer disease develops silently over many years before causing any symptoms. Consequently, some people's brains might tolerate and adapt to a greater degree of disease before any symptoms appear. Or, maybe, if two people had the same amount of Alzheimer disease in their brains, the one with more cognitive reserve would have fewer or no symptoms. Someone with higher cognitive reserve is more likely to be diagnosed with dementia when the Alzheimer disease in their brain is at an advanced stage. As such, they may decline faster following diagnosis.

But what influences cognitive reserve? As we know, factors from all life stages – even before birth – affect us. The same is true of cognitive reserve: education in early life, socioeconomic position, nutrition, illness, our occupation later in life, and lifestyle factors like engaging in cognitively stimulating activities and aerobic exercise. It seems that, rather than being fixed, our cognitive reserve is modifiable over our lifetime. This is a hopeful message, just like the one that says it is never too late to think about optimizing our dementia risk.

How do memory and thinking skills change as one ages?

Some abilities, such as processing speed and reaction time, decline as we age. Aged 80, most people find that they cannot react as quickly as in their prime. Vocabulary and wisdom increase and remain at their peak for most people, even into later life. However, memory tends not to decline in healthy ageing. As a result, memory problems should be looked into but, importantly, do not always mean dementia.

3

How can I reduce my risk of developing dementia?

Is dementia preventable?

There is not a straightforward answer to this question. Even the word 'prevent' is problematic. First, it suggests that someone who develops dementia has somehow failed to stop their dementia or is to blame for their illness. Second, because the disease which results in dementia starts in midlife, we are not talking about 'preventing' dementia but about delaying or stopping the symptoms of Alzheimer disease. And finally, it is more accurate to speak of 'risk reduction' rather than 'prevention'. For example, should you stop smoking or improve your diet so you don't develop diabetes, this will also change your subsequent risk of dementia. In short, everyone can reduce their risk of dementia, but it is impossible to prevent dementia completely. You can't reduce the risk of developing dementia to zero.

Is what's good for the heart good for the brain?

There is a lot of overlap between the risk factors for dementia and known risk factors for heart disease – high blood pressure (hypertension), obesity, smoking and diabetes. So, if you stop smoking, for instance, this will help your cardiovascular system, lower your risk of heart disease, and reduce your risk of developing dementia.

One obvious way in which what is good for the heart is good for the head is vascular dementia. This dementia is the result of the lifelong process of cardiovascular disease affecting the circulation of the body, leading to angina, ischaemic heart disease, and heart attacks. The process also damages blood vessels within the brain. Over time, this can lead to a stroke (if a large vessel becomes blocked), transient ischaemic attacks (temporary mini-strokes), or vascular dementia.

Does alcohol cause dementia?

Alcohol is a poison, albeit one used in medicinal quantities in many cultures for thousands of years. Alcohol can be harmful to the brain, and not only to people who have an alcohol 'problem'.

The technical term for addiction is dependence. In the case of alcohol, a person becomes tolerant and so must drink more to get the same effect. They continue to drink excessively despite recognizing the difficulties it causes. They then begin to have withdrawal effects – for instance, shaking in the morning – leading them to drink more. In this process, their body is becoming physically dependent on alcohol.

People who use alcohol excessively – enough to damage their health – but are not dependent are called 'harmful users'. A large percentage of the population falls into this category as they drink more than the recommended 14 units of alcohol per week, with several alcohol-free days.

However, even people who consume an average amount of alcohol over an extended period can develop cognitive problems, which ultimately can become dementia. The result is alcohol-related brain damage. Stopping drinking – which, if you drink a lot, should be done gradually – can stabilize cognitive decline. Although there might be some slight cognitive improvement, once it is present, alcohol-related brain damage is, basically, irreversible.

A person with a severe alcohol problem absorbs fewer vitamins and minerals from their diet, which might already lack nutritional value. One possible effect of long-term alcohol use is the Wernicke–Korsakoff syndrome, resulting from a deficiency of vitamin B1 (thiamine). Symptoms include difficulties walking (ataxia), confusion, and alterations in eye movements (ophthalmoplegia). Untreated, it can progress to (the usually irreversible) Korsakoff syndrome. A person with Korsakoff syndrome can experience amnesia, especially an inability to learn new memories. They might also confabulate, which means they can fluently (but not deliberately) make up stories or explanations to fill gaps in their memory.

If you are worried about your drinking, you should consult your doctor before making any changes yourself. Suddenly stopping drinking alcohol at substantial levels can be dangerous. If you want to find out more, there are helpful online resources, such as

Are head injuries linked to dementia?

There is significant popular interest in the potential link between mild head injuries ('concussion') sustained in sports – such as football, rugby, or boxing – and dementia. Such head injuries are unlikely to be good for your brain. However, in most people, even regular concussions are unlikely to be the only potential cause of dementia, and it is not the case that everyone who played football and rugby will develop dementia.

What about hearing loss?

Hearing loss is common, particularly as we get older. Hearing loss in midlife is associated with increased dementia risk, but the relationship is unclear. However, using a hearing aid for hearing difficulties can improve communication, help promote social engagement, and reduce the risk of delirium.

Am I too late to reduce my risk of dementia?

When Tom sees someone in his clinic who smokes, he enthusiastically tells them that there is never a time in life when you are too late to stop smoking. It is always the healthiest decision you can make.

The situation with other risk factors is not so clear. Figure 3.1 shows the main risk factors for dementia. It shows that, over a lifetime, different risk (or protective) factors take effect at different points. Most people complete most of their education relatively early in life, at school and, possibly, college or university. So, by middle age, it is too late to change how long you spent at school as a child. However, remaining intellectually stimulated through your work and interests is important.

The brain is more sensitive to the effects of high blood pressure in midlife than at other times. This might explain why it is in midlife that high blood pressure and obesity seem to have the most effect on dementia risk. Keeping your blood pressure under control later in life has beneficial health impacts without specifically affecting your dementia risk.

Changing your lifestyle is likely to benefit your overall health, even if it might not always influence your dementia risk:

- Maintain a healthy weight.
- Avoid developing diabetes (or keep it well controlled if you have developed it).
- Stop smoking.
- Keep blood pressure under control.
- Don't drink too much.
- Keep physically and socially active.

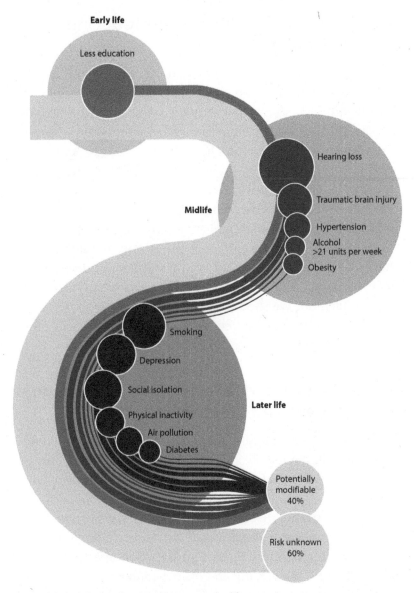

Figure 3.1 Risk factors for dementia across the life course
The size of the circles next to each risk factor shows the relative importance of each one.

Adapted with permission from G. Livingston et al. (2020), Dementia prevention, intervention, and care: 2020 report of the Lancet Commission, *Lancet 396:* P413–46. https://doi.org/10.1016/S0140-6736(20)30367-6

Am I too early to think about reducing my risk of dementia?

In a radio interview, Tom once said, 'It is never too early to think about reducing your risk of dementia.' A colleague who had heard him pointed out that the point of conception was presumably too early for him to think about this! Yes – but also, no. Clearly, when Tom was a fertilized egg, he wasn't in a position to do anything. Still, some of his dementia risk was already in place. As we saw above, genetic factors influence his dementia risk, and he inherited these genes from his parents. His experiences in the womb and very early in life also impacted his dementia risk. Dementia risk is not only modifiable – we have the power to affect our risk of developing dementia, at least partially – but the factors that are active early in life are very influential. We should all encourage our children, nieces, nephews, and grandchildren to complete as much education as possible!

What about the risk factors we can change – environment and lifestyle?

Air pollution has received a great deal of attention in recent years. It is now believed that exposure to air pollution – commonly the result of traffic – harms many aspects of human health, including dementia.

We understand the direct and indirect ways air pollution influences cardiovascular disease risk. While we don't yet have a similar understanding of how air pollution affects the brain, the evidence is convincing and overwhelming.

There is even evidence that air pollution particles get into the brain. The brain is generally well protected by the blood–brain barrier keeping unwanted things out. These particles, however, have managed to pass through this barrier into the brain. More detail about the relationship between air pollution and dementia can be found in the Alzheimer's Society report 'Is there a link between air pollution and dementia?'

Physical activity is important throughout life, but particularly in later life for dementia risk. You don't need to run marathons or compete in triathlons. About half an hour of moderate exercise (walking, for example) daily is enough. If you aren't active at all, making a gentle start is a sensible change.

Social activity also affects dementia risk. Try to keep socially engaged and avoid becoming isolated. One thing we learned from the coronavirus pandemic is that human beings need community. Many people become more isolated as they get older, as friends and relatives move away or die. Taking steps to remain connected and make new friends could be vital.

Many people ask about brain training, crosswords, and other puzzles. There is nothing wrong with these activities, but the evidence suggests that, while doing puzzles and crosswords might make you better at them, they do little to improve other cognitive skills.

What about risk factors we can't change: genetic ones, for example?

People who have inherited one or more copies of a particular gene from their parents are at an increased risk of developing dementia compared to others. However, these days the focus is no longer on the idea of a 'gene for' something. Instead, most conditions, dementia included, are influenced by very large numbers of genes, all of which have tiny effects on increasing or decreasing your risk. The sum of these tiny effects gives you a 'polygenic risk score' unique to you, which will explain more about your dementia risk than any single gene. (For further information about modern genetics and polygenic risk scores, we recommend *The Gene: An Intimate History* by Siddhartha

Mukherjee [Scribner 2016] and *Blueprint: How DNA Makes Us Who We Are* [Penguin, 2018] by Robert Plomin.)

We can't change our genetic makeup, and if you were participating in a research study, you wouldn't be told about your genotype. These days, though, you can order a kit to collect your saliva to send away to have your genotype analysed. It tells you your polygenic risk score for many things – including Alzheimer disease, body mass index, depression, and so on – in addition to specific genes. Knowing this won't allow you to change your genes, but some people find learning about their genetic risk of dementia motivates them to optimize their risk in the areas they can change – for example, by stopping smoking, drinking less alcohol, or being more physically and socially active.

4

What are the most common types of dementia?

What is Alzheimer dementia?

Alzheimer disease is the most common cause of dementia. Typically, someone with Alzheimer dementia presents with memory difficulties, especially short-term memory. People notice difficulties finding words or people's names, remembering where they have put things, and repeating questions or stories. These memory problems often develop gradually and are usually more noticeable to friends and relatives than to the person themself.

Memory difficulties get worse over time, and, eventually, other thinking skills become affected. The person's ability to carry out daily activities independently will be impacted. Clinically, Alzheimer dementia is a diagnosis of exclusion; there cannot be any other potential cause in evidence. The doctor might suggest a CT or MRI scan to show any shrinkage in the brain. It is possible to identify Alzheimer disease (but not Alzheimer dementia) using a PET scan, but this is not currently used in clinical practice.

Over time, Alzheimer dementia symptoms become increasingly noticeable, and the person becomes more reliant on others for support. Ultimately, depending on their individual care needs and the support their carers can provide, it may no longer be possible to support them at home.

What is vascular dementia?

The second most common cause of dementia is disease in the blood vessels in the brain – the same process which affects circulation elsewhere in the body leading to cardiovascular disease. These changes result in three changes in the brain:

- strokes which cause noticeable and more or less permanent symptoms
- small 'silent' strokes which don't cause noticeable symptoms, but may cause more subtle changes over time
- restriction of oxygen to brain cells over an extended period.

People with vascular dementia present with various cognitive symptoms and might be aware of the changes they are experiencing. This can be very upsetting and is a different experience from Alzheimer dementia where the person is often unaware of their memory problems from quite an early stage.

What is mixed dementia?

Both Alzheimer disease and vascular changes are common and can occur together. Someone may present with a history and investigations showing evidence of an Alzheimer-type picture and some aspects that point towards vascular dementia. Such a patient would probably be told that they have mixed dementia – that is, the dementia syndrome with likely both Alzheimer and vascular processes underlying it.

The older a person is, the more likely they are to have multiple illnesses. In the same way, as someone ages, their brain will accumulate conditions. In someone of advanced age, it is likely that several different factors cause dementia.

What is dementia with Lewy bodies?

Dementia with Lewy bodies is the third most common cause of dementia, affecting at least one in 20 people with dementia (and possibly as many as one in five). Symptoms include:

- fluctuating cognition (varying over a single day rather than good days and bad days)
- visual hallucinations (often animals or small children)
- REM sleep behaviour disorder (vivid dreams in association with active movements when asleep)
- symptoms of parkinsonism (slow movements, rigidity, and tremor).

This type of dementia is generally underdiagnosed because symptoms vary, change, and evolve.

What is Parkinson disease dementia?

The same process in the brain causes dementia with Lewy bodies and Parkinson disease, and someone with Parkinson disease may develop dementia later in their illness.

What are the frontotemporal dementias?

Rarer dementias that particularly affect the front part of the brain have been recognized for many years. Pick disease, for instance, was first described by Dr Arnold Pick (1854–1924), a Czech doctor, in 1892. The frontotemporal dementias include behavioural variant frontotemporal dementia and primary progressive aphasia. These conditions can present earlier than other dementias, and memory might remain relatively intact in the early stages.

Behavioural variant frontotemporal dementia often shows changes in personality or behaviour. There can be a loss of inhibitions resulting in out-of-character behaviour. Other features include apathy or inertia, increasingly rigid habits or the adoption of rituals, and sometimes a preference for sweet foods.

There are two types of primary progressive aphasias, and both involve marked changes in language use and understanding. Not being able to express yourself can be very frustrating, and the resulting communication difficulties can present significant challenges for the person and their family.

What is LATE?

LATE – limbic-predominant age-associated TDP-43 encephalopathy – is a brain disease only identified in 2019. It leads to similar symptoms to Alzheimer dementia. LATE can coexist with Alzheimer disease as well as other conditions. We are at a very early stage in our understanding of this disease, and it reminds us of how complex the brain is and how far we are from fully understanding it.

5

Are there other conditions that look like dementia?

Depression and anxiety

Many people Tom sees in his memory clinic have memory problems but do not have dementia. Instead, a good proportion are experiencing anxiety and/or depression. Depression is an illness – a common and treatable one – which, the textbooks say, is characterized by at least two of the following three symptoms: low mood, reduced energy, and decreased activity.

However, the textbooks aren't always correct. Many older people Tom has seen with depression wouldn't describe their mood as low, saying, 'But I don't *feel* depressed.' Instead, feeling 'fed up' better describes how they feel. Other features of depression include a reduced ability to enjoy or to get pleasure from things, feelings of guilt, disturbed sleep, poor appetite, and decreased interest in sex.

Some dementias are characterized by apathy or tiredness, which can sometimes be difficult to distinguish from depression. The more psychological features – such as not being able to get pleasure from things or feeling guilty – can help to identify the problem as depression.

Someone who is depressed can also experience memory difficulties – and will score poorly on cognitive testing – because they lack the motivation to make a cognitive effort. Rather than getting the answers wrong, someone who is depressed often answers 'I don't know' repeatedly during a memory test.

Anxiety is also common and often goes together with depression. Some people say that they have always been 'a worrier', and, undoubtedly, there are those who worry about things more than others. However, when anxiety becomes a real problem, someone can spend most of the time preoccupied with their anxious thoughts. This experience of being constantly distracted means that they can ignore what is happening around them and might not register conversations or information told to them. As such, they might not be able to recall them later. While anxiety can appear like a memory problem, then, it isn't the same thing.

Despite what many people think, both anxiety and depression are treatable conditions. Treatment should be organized by your GP (family doctor or primary care physician) or, if necessary, a specialist like a psychiatrist. The main treatments are talking therapies and medication, which work well together. Talking therapies include counselling, cognitive behavioural therapy (CBT), interpersonal psychotherapy (IPT), and psychodynamic/psychoanalytic psychotherapy. They can involve seeing a counsellor or therapist once a week (or more often) to talk about yourself and your symptoms. Access to talking therapies can vary and may involve a financial commitment.

Medication prescribed for depression and anxiety is often an antidepressant. These are very effective medications and tend not to cause many side effects. However, as with tranquillizers like benzodiazepines (diazepam and related drugs), you should take them only under medical advice.

Some people find that alcohol helps their anxiety. However, relying on alcohol can cause significant health problems and might result in memory problems in its own right. We would therefore encourage you to seek professional help with your anxiety instead.

Infection

When humans become unwell – with an infection, for example – they respond in a stereotypical way. Doctors use the word 'delirium' to describe this reaction, which is characterized by confusion, disorientation in time and place, and sometimes hallucinations or delusions. It can be very distressing for the person experiencing it and their family, not least because sometimes people behave bizarrely or entirely out of character. While this can happen at any age, older people are more likely to respond to an illness by developing delirium and can take some time to recover. The cognitive symptoms of delirium resemble dementia, but the timescale is usually more rapid – over days to weeks rather than months or years.

Nutritional

Vitamin deficiencies – particularly vitamins B12 and B9 (folate) – can be associated with memory problems. A blood test to check vitamin levels (among other things) is one of the first things your doctor will suggest when you speak with them about your memory. Should you be deficient in one or more of these vitamins, your doctor will recommend tablets and/or injections as a replacement.

Hormonal

Another test your doctor will arrange is your thyroid function. Your thyroid gland, which is in your neck, can be overactive or underactive. In the latter case – if you are hypothyroid – the level of thyroid hormone in your body is too low. You might find that you feel tired, gain weight, feel low in mood, and your memory is not as good as it was. All these symptoms can improve if you take replacement thyroid hormone to normalize your levels.

Many women experience changes in memory during menopause, and there is some evidence that the hormone oestrogen may have a protective effect on the brain. Whether or not hormone replacement therapy (HRT) is associated with a reduced risk of developing dementia is not currently clear. The possible benefits of using HRT must be weighed against the known risks.

Medication side effects

When a doctor prescribes a medication, they weigh the potential benefits against possible side effects or harms. Tom tries to involve his patient in this discussion and, as far as possible, seek their views on this decision. However, in some cases, a medication might have been prescribed a long time ago and never been reviewed or stopped. It was initially appropriate and unlikely to cause side effects. However, several years later, it might have started to cause problems. The balance between benefits and harms changes over time and with age.

Many drugs have unintended consequences on a chemical neurotransmitter in the brain. One example is the drug solifenacin (trade name: Vesicare), frequently prescribed for urinary frequency or incontinence. The appropriateness of solifenacin should be reviewed every three to six months, but this doesn't always happen. It is not uncommon for someone to end up on this medication for years. Over time, it can start to have a detrimental effect on the brain, often resulting in some memory problems. We have seen some people transformed by stopping this medication, but others stop and find their memory problems do not change. However, you won't know without trying. As always, we advise you not to change anything without discussing it with your doctor.

Other neurological causes

A further condition to rule out when someone presents with memory problems is normal-pressure hydrocephalus, or excess fluid within the brain, which can show on a brain scan. It is usually associated with difficulties walking, urinary symptoms, and memory problems. An operation can sometimes help.

6

How is dementia diagnosed?

Should I speak to my GP about my memory?

If you, your family or your friends are concerned about your memory, it would be sensible to contact your GP. However, don't jump to the conclusion that you are developing dementia. Dementia is a possibility, not a certainty.

An assessment might identify a progressive illness like dementia or a treatable/reversible condition like medication side effects or depression and anxiety.

You could be diagnosed with 'mild cognitive impairment' (relatively minor memory difficulties that do not interfere with daily activities). You can recover from mild cognitive impairment. You can also remain stable, or it can progress to dementia.

Even if the assessment concludes that your memory is currently OK, it can help to have a baseline measurement of your memory and other cognitive abilities should you experience a change in the future.

How important is early diagnosis of dementia?

The timing of a dementia diagnosis is significant. An 'early' diagnosis maximizes the benefits of post-diagnostic information, support, and medication. It can help you remain independent for as long as possible.

On the other hand, a consultant must be confident they are making the correct diagnosis. Should a person present with relatively minor memory problems, it is not always easy to determine whether they have early dementia or mild cognitive impairment. To some extent, it is a judgement based on expectations of what older people should be able to do.

Many people told they have a mild cognitive impairment find that their memory improves over time. Moreover, a person with a mild cognitive impairment treated with dementia medication (cholinesterase inhibitors) will experience none of the benefits but many side effects, such as nausea, diarrhoea, muscle cramps, and nightmares

For this reason, the phrase 'timely diagnosis' is increasingly popular. It removes the possible inference that a diagnosis has been made too early – that is, before it is certain that the diagnosis is correct. 'Timely diagnosis' is used in Alzheimer Europe's Glasgow Declaration in 2014.

The Glasgow Declaration of 2014 (<www.alzheimer-europe.org/policy/campaign/glasgow-declaration-2014>) affirms that every person living with dementia has the right to:

- a timely diagnosis
- access to quality post-diagnostic support
- person-centred, coordinated, quality care throughout their illness
- equitable access to treatments and therapeutic interventions
- be respected as an individual in their community.

How do I get referred for memory assessment?

Health service structures vary across the world, but if you are worried about your memory, the first point of contact is usually your GP or family doctor. In some places, you might be able to refer yourself to a memory clinic or specialist (neurologist/geriatrician/psychiatrist) directly. Here, we will describe the process in the UK National Health Service, where your GP is the first point of contact.

If you are worried about your memory, you can make an appointment to see your GP in the usual way. Your GP will ask you questions and to complete a brief pencil and paper test of your memory and other thinking skills. They will also arrange blood tests and, possibly, a brain scan.

If your GP feels that further assessment is needed, he or she will then make a referral for a memory assessment, which can take place in a clinic or your own home. In the UK, your GP will refer you to the old age (geriatric) psychiatry service. Many people are surprised by this, believing they are neither old nor in need of psychiatry. In other countries, you may see a neurologist or a geriatrician. Still, the approach taken will be similar regardless of the kind of doctor you see.

Who should be referred for memory assessment?

Anyone worried about their memory or who has noticed a change in their memory should consult their doctor. The doctor will run some tests and identify if there is anything treatable. They might also refer you for further memory assessment by a specialist service, sometimes called a memory clinic.

Importantly, not everyone referred to a memory clinic ends up with a diagnosis of dementia. A clinic can identify people who do not have dementia and, if appropriate, start treatment for the non-dementia cause of their memory problems.

What if my relative refuses to see a doctor about their memory?

Particularly in Alzheimer dementia, changes in a person's memory are often more noticeable to others than to them. As a relative, you might notice your relative repeating themselves, asking the same questions, or muddling up appointments. However, when you raise your concerns, they might deny there is anything wrong and even become irritated or hostile. Consequently, there might be a long delay between first noticing a change in your relative's memory and being seen by their doctor.

While a doctor will usually not discuss a patient's care with someone else without consent (even a family member or next of kin), they can listen. It can help to contact your relative's doctor to make them aware of your concerns about their memory. An opportunity to discuss memory might present itself if the person attends for another reason. If required, a referral to a memory clinic can then follow.

When meeting Tom in the clinic, it is not unusual for someone to be oblivious to their memory problems. Should it become clear that a diagnosis of dementia is appropriate, a decision needs to be made about how best to tell the person. It is almost always the right thing to do to tell someone the diagnosis. They might disagree, but it means identifying what is going on and exploring what might help. Tom is surprised by how many people who strongly disagree with his diagnosis of dementia are nevertheless happy to take medication to help their memory.

Very rarely, should the harm outweigh the benefits of giving a diagnosis, Tom would not explicitly tell the person about their diagnosis. However, he would propose the same management plan and support.

Why am I asked to do so many (cognitive) tests?

The two components of the dementia syndrome are: (1) progressive cognitive impairment; (2) which impacts the person's day-to-day functioning. The reason for asking you to do so many cognitive tests is to back up your account of memory changes with an objective measurement. Depending on the context, different tests are required. For rapid memory screening – for example, when a person is admitted to a hospital – there are several brief tests, including the Abbreviated Mental Test.

More detailed screening tests can clarify if a person present-ing to their doctor should be referred for further memory assess-ment. These tests include the 'Mini-Mental State Examination' or the 'Montreal Cognitive Assessment'.

At the memory assessment itself, you will usually be asked to complete a more extensive test such as 'Addenbrooke's Cognitive Examination'. All these tests are very similar and focus on various skills (or domains, such as memory, orienta-tion, and visuospatial abilities) in more or less detail.

Some people might also be referred to a clinical psychologist for neuropsychological testing. Such testing can take several hours – usually spread over multiple appointments – but can provide a detailed picture of your strengths and the difficul-ties you are experiencing. Neuropsychological testing can be additional evidence to guide a decision about whether your memory problems are early dementia or not. The process can be especially helpful if a person is very bright and likely to per-form well on cognitive tests, even if they have some cognitive impairment.

Should I have a brain scan?

The UK National Institute of Health and Care Excellence (NICE) advises that everyone should be offered structural brain imaging (usually a computed tomography [CT] or magnetic resonance imaging [MRI] scan) during the process of memory assessment unless it is clear that the person has dementia and what the subtype is. A scan aims to identify any reversible causes for the memory problem or to help clarify the subtype.

A CT scan uses X-rays to image the brain and involves exposure to a small amount of radiation. While small, it is approximately the same as having 100 chest X-rays or the annual background radiation to which people in the UK are exposed. MRI, on the other hand, uses magnets rather than radiation and produces a more detailed image of your brain.

It is important to remember that a brain scan alone cannot diagnose dementia. It is better to think of it as one piece of the jigsaw puzzle of memory assessment.

What is a biomarker?

You might hear the word 'biomarker' in relation to memory assessment. Biomarker is short for *bio*logical *marker* and can refer to brain scans, certain blood tests, or lumbar puncture (spinal tap). All are used in research, but only brain scans are routinely used in clinical practice.

What will happen when I am assessed?

We know some things about ourselves that no one else knows, so we are the only person to ask. However, there are also some things about ourselves we are unaware of, but other people can report. For this reason, you will usually be invited to bring someone with you who knows you well to provide a collateral history.

You and the person accompanying you will be asked about the development of your memory problems and any associated difficulties. You will also be asked about your daily activities and any need for support. You will usually be asked several other questions about your medical history, childhood education and occupation, among other topics.

You will also be asked to complete a pencil-and-paper cognitive assessment, which can be a little daunting. Some people feel they are back in school and worry they might fail the test. (Franz Kafka said that we spend the first part of our lives taking tests to get into institutions and the later part taking tests to keep out of them.) However, this is not the purpose of the tests. Their job is to give objective evidence to complement the history you provided. They can highlight areas of strength and the difficulties you are experiencing.

It might be possible to gather enough information from one appointment to come to a conclusion, or your doctor might suggest further investigations, such as a brain scan. Sometimes it can also be helpful to allow some time to pass to see any changes or whether things remain stable.

If required, the doctor should tell you clearly but sensitively about your dementia diagnosis and give you time to ask questions. If offered medication, you should be given enough information to help decide if you want to try it. You should be told who will follow up with you and how you can contact them with any questions or problems. You might also want to find out what research is happening in your area and how to get involved.

7

I've been diagnosed with dementia

What should I do next?

Every person given a diagnosis of dementia reacts differently. Some might have felt apprehensive about attending the appointment and not be able to take it all in. For others, it can be a relief that, after an exhaustive (and sometimes exhausting) assessment, there is a diagnosis to explain their difficulties. They can begin to plan to maximize their quality of life from now on.

Another reason to have someone you trust at the appointment is that they can also listen and support you in asking questions.

Your doctor will likely provide you with further information to take away and read – about the illness, support and treatments, and local research opportunities. It might feel overwhelming, and you don't need to read everything straight away or tackle every potential issue in advance. Each person adapts to the reality of the diagnosis at their speed. Dementia doesn't have to become the defining fact of your life from now on.

In Scotland, where we both work, the National Dementia Strategy states that everyone diagnosed with dementia is entitled to at least one year of post-diagnostic support from a named professional. Alzheimer Scotland's 'Five Pillars Model of Post-Diagnostic Support' (Figure 7.1) outlines how this support aims to help people diagnosed with dementia and their families to live as well as possible and prepare for the future. This approach can improve the initial experience of living with dementia and reduce the need for care services.

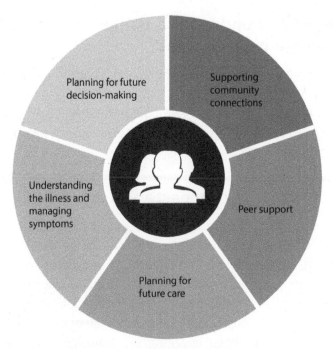

Figure 7.1 Alzheimer Scotland's Five Pillars Model of Post-Diagnostic Support

While this model is not used everywhere, the principles are universal. By the end of the first year, the person and their family will have produced a personal plan incorporating their natural supports. They will have developed new peer support mechanisms alongside existing and new community connections. They will hopefully be in a better position to live independently with dementia for as long as possible.

Post-diagnostic support must be personalized and flexible, responding to individual needs. Some people want to engage immediately, while others need more time to adjust to the diagnosis before accepting support. Others might never wish to receive support.

1 How can I understand dementia and manage its symptoms?

The first pillar is about supporting you and your family to come to terms with the diagnosis and learn to self-manage the condition. It involves your family and your natural support networks as the main source of support, moving away from a hierarchical patient–professional model.

2 How can I stay connected to my community?

To enhance your quality of life and increase the support you receive from those around you, you should be supported to maintain, reconnect with and build on your existing social networks. This can help avoid isolation and may reduce the need for care services in the future. This 'risk-enabling' approach allows you to take appropriate risks with a safety net to help you remain an active citizen engaging in meaningful mainstream community activities.

3 Would peer support from other people with dementia help?

Peer support can help you come to terms with the illness, try new strategies for coping with adversity, maintain your well-being and develop resilience. Peer support can provide positive examples of living well with dementia and encourage you and your family to weigh the benefits of independence against the risks. Talking openly and honestly with people experiencing similar challenges builds bonds and can help with negative emotions such as frustration.

4 Should I plan future decision-making?

It is important to make informed choices about your future while you can. You can arrange powers of attorney and formally state your wishes about your finances and future care and treatment. Understanding your local systems can help you know when and how to access relevant support from health and social care.

5 Can I plan the shape of my future care?

You could develop a personal plan setting out your choices, hopes and aspirations for the future. You should always be at the centre of this plan, which should be a living document based on your strengths. Doing this can help you think creatively about the support you require and how the people around you can be a positive part of that support. It should include a series of goals, steps, and outcomes that your supporters will help you to realize. You can also use this opportunity to record your life story.

8

How is dementia treated?

Is there a cure for dementia? Can the disease process be reversed?

Many people think there is little that can help someone with dementia. Although there are only a few effective treatments, they can make a small but noticeable difference. Timely, high-quality post-diagnostic information and support are also important. So, while we may not currently have a cure or be able to reverse the disease process, appropriate support and treatment do help.

Are there medications available to treat dementia? What do they do?

The medications we have to treat dementia treat the symptoms rather than 'curing' the underlying illness or altering the course of the disease. There are two groups of medications – cholinesterase inhibitors and memantine.

Medication	Trade name(s)
Cholinesterase inhibitors	
donepezil	Aricept, Adlarity
rivastigmine	Exelon
galantamine	Acumor, Consion, Gaalin, Galsya, Galzemic, Gatalin, Lotprosin, Luventa, Razadyne, Reminyl
Memantine	Axura, Ebixa, Marixino, Namenda, Valios

Cholinesterase inhibitors

Cholinesterase inhibitors boost the effects of acetylcholine, one of the chemical messengers our brain cells use to communicate. These medicines are not transformative but benefit about two-thirds of people who take them. Memory decline can slow down or even pause for a few months. People can retain abilities, remain more independent, and live at home longer. There is also evidence that these medicines have subtle positive effects in the longer term. Like many treatments (for high blood pressure or diabetes, for example), you are likely to be advised to continue taking it for the rest of your life.

Memantine

Memantine works differently from cholinesterase inhibitors. It reduces the excitability of our brain cells by blocking the action of glutamate, another chemical messenger. Glutamate is one of various chemical messengers and it has an 'excitatory' effect on those brain cells receiving its signals. Memantine blocks this effect.

What about aducanumab or lecanemab?

There was worldwide excitement in 2021 when the US Federal Drug Administration approved aducanumab (Aduhelm) under the accelerated approval pathway, which is used when a drug's benefits are uncertain. Evidence for the benefits of aducanumab was mixed, and it has not been approved in the rest of the world.

At the time of writing, there is similar excitement about summary results of another potential new treatment, lecanemab. Two further trials – of gantenerumab and donanemab – are due to report in the near future. We are hopeful that an effective treatment for Alzheimer dementia may be available in the medium term. But nothing is certain and the full results are not public yet, so it is unknown if any of these treatments will ultimately be licensed for use.

Should I take vitamins or supplements?

Many people take multivitamins or dietary supplements, but there is no evidence that their general usage reduces the risk of dementia or slows its progression.

However, should you be deficient in a particular vitamin, your doctor will probably recommend you take vitamins to replenish your levels. A deficiency in vitamins B12 or B9 (folate) may cause memory problems which look like early dementia.

Many people are deficient in vitamin D, which comes from our diet and sunlight stimulating our skin to produce it. Levels of the vitamin vary depending on the time of year, with most people having less in winter. Levels stay low for longer the further you are from the equator. At higher latitudes, the sun is also sometimes not strong enough to stimulate our bodies to produce vitamin D. Vitamin D deficiency is linked to an increased risk of developing dementia. However, we don't currently know if replacing vitamin D (by taking supplements or enriching foods) can reduce the risk.

What non-medical interventions are available?

Many lifestyle and care-based therapies can help people with dementia. They are used in a variety of settings and for different reasons. Some approaches seem to work in the community but not in care homes. Some seem to work to improve quality of life but not on symptoms such as agitation. It's worth trying a range of approaches to find out what works for the person. Unfortunately, not all therapies are available everywhere.

The approach taken most often with people with dementia is person-centred care. In this approach, every intervention and treatment choice should be informed by an in-depth under-standing of the person, what makes them tick, and the experi-ences they have had throughout their life.

Other approaches used with people with dementia include behavioural therapy, reality orientation, validation therapy, reminiscence therapy, coping strategy-based family carer ther-apy, art therapy, activity therapies (including dance, movement, drama, etc.), complementary therapies such as aromatherapy, light therapy, and multi-sensory approaches (such as Snoezelen multi-sensory environments).

What is cognitive stimulation therapy?

The UK National Institute of Health and Care Excellence (NICE) recommends cognitive stimulation therapy (CST) for people with mild to moderate dementia. Instead of focusing on cog-nition, the person with dementia identifies the functional goals that are important to them. CST works with the person's strengths and attempts to compensate for any areas of difficulty to help them achieve these goals.

Is music helpful?

Music is a vital part of life for many people. Over and above sty-listic preferences – whether you would choose Orthodox chant over the latest number one – music is associated with significant memories for many people. We also know that music involves multiple brain areas and is relatively protected against dementia-related changes. It can be recognized and affect people even with quite advanced dementia. Music therapy is a specialized treatment that can be run as a group or with individuals and can greatly benefit people with dementia.

Music can also be used in less specialized ways. Several organizations – including Playlist for Life, Music and Memory, and Music for My Mind – advocate using personally meaning-ful music as a treatment for people with dementia. This means music associated with specific memories and personal stories: the first dance at your wedding, the music you always played driving to the countryside on holiday, the theme music for the *Eurovision Song Contest*...!

Many family members and carers find certain pieces of music provoke recognition and even brief moments of transformation for people with dementia. They can give a sense of connection which had been missing. Playlist for Life and the other organi-zations mentioned above have many moving stories and videos on their websites demonstrating the enormous value of music for someone with dementia.

9

Should I take part in research?

What is research?

'Research' is a word that often puts people off, thinking of it as something that only special people do. Increasingly, however, the vital contribution of people with 'lived experience' to research is being recognized.

Taking part in research does not have to be demanding, time-consuming or painful. At its heart, research tries to answer questions and further our understanding of the world. How it goes about this depends on the specific questions being asked, which determine the type of research carried out and the experience of taking part.

The two main types of research are quantitative and qualitative. However, many projects include elements of both – mixed-methods research.

- **Quantitative research** seeks to measure things and often involves numbers. The questions it seeks to answer usually start with 'how much' or 'how often' – for example: *How many people with diabetes develop dementia? How much does having a particular genetic variant increase your risk of dementia? How often do doctors ask their patients if they have any questions during a memory clinic appointment?*
- **Qualitative research**, on the other hand, seeks to understand things and usually involves interviews or focus groups, sometimes with questions and prompts, but sometimes just a simple conversation. Qualitative researchers might be interested in: *What did it feel like to be diagnosed with dementia? What makes you feel freer when you have dementia?*

Both types of research – quantitative and qualitative – are complementary, and neither is better than the other. Which you use depends on what question you are trying to answer.

What sort of research can people with dementia participate in?

The most straightforward type of research to take part in is a questionnaire or an interview. A researcher interested in some aspect of your experience will ask questions or have a conversation with you. Sometimes the researchers might ask you to participate in a focus group, which is an interview with several people simultaneously. These interviews or focus groups can be one-off, or there might be a series of them.

Another type of research is a cohort study, which follows a group of people over time to see how things change for them. The participants usually have something in common: all being born in the same year or living in the same area, for instance. These studies are almost always observational. The researchers will ask you questions and take physical measurements, perhaps with blood tests and scans, but will not give you a treatment. They are only interested in how things change over time and, often, if there is anything particular about you that can predict what might happen to you in the future.

Sometimes, observational studies are cross-sectional, which means they see people only at one point in time. They range from studies which take various measurements and investigations to studies which look at only one thing.

Another option available to people with dementia is pledging to donate brain tissue for research purposes after you die. In the UK, you can register with Brains for Dementia Research (in England and Wales) or the Alzheimer Scotland Dementia Brain Tissue Bank run by the University of Edinburgh (in Scotland).

A final type of research is a clinical trial of a new treatment or intervention, which could be administered as a tablet, an infusion through a drip, or some other kind of treatment. A trial can require a long-term commitment (often two or three years) to attend the hospital regularly for cognitive assessments, physical checks, and blood tests, and, sometimes, to receive the treatment under study.

Most clinical trials are placebo-controlled, meaning the active treatment is compared to an inactive sugar pill. You would be randomly selected to receive either the treatment or the placebo, and no one in the research team would know which you were receiving until the end of the trial. In other words, you might participate in the trial and not receive the treatment. However, this is essential to determine if the treatment works.

Some trials study brand-new treatments we know little about, and some study treatments already licensed and used for other conditions that may have an effect on dementia. In the latter case, we know much more about the treatment and its safety, whereas in the case of a new treatment, less is known, so the risks are slightly greater.

Should I be concerned about taking part in research?

To ensure it is carried out safely and ethically, any research conducted by a reputable body, such as a university or healthcare system (e.g. the NHS in the UK), is subject to rules and regulations. An independent ethics committee must approve all research.

The research team should provide you with the information and time you need to make an informed decision about participating in their research. You should never feel pressured to take part, and, importantly, even if you do decide to take part in a study, you are always free to withdraw at any point. You don't need to give a reason.

If you have concerns about how the research you are participating in is being conducted, you have several options:

- You can speak with the research team or, in the case of large, international trials, the organization in charge of the study.
- When consenting to take part, you will have been given the name of an independent contact with whom you can share your concerns.
- In the NHS, there is the usual NHS complaints procedure, which also applies to research conducted in the NHS.
- Research conducted by for-profit research organizations is subject to the same ethical requirements as research conducted within the NHS (or other healthcare settings). While they are still required to comply with international standards of Good Clinical Practice, they are subject to different governance procedures than NHS researchers.
- Finally, you can make a specific complaint against any practitioner or researcher you feel is not practising as they should. For example, you can report a doctor in the UK to the General Medical Council, which registers and licenses all doctors.

How can I find out what research is happening?

Your nurse or doctor (the specialists or your GP) should be able to tell you about research happening locally. They may even have leaflets or posters on display in their waiting rooms. Dementia charities – there is a list at the end of the book – will also be able to link you with ongoing research in your area.

Another way to find out about research opportunities near you is to join a research interest register. In the UK, *Join Dementia Research* is a database you can sign up to for this purpose. You will then be linked to studies you might be eligible for and can opt to be contacted by the researchers to find out more. In Scotland, the NHS Research Scotland Neuroprogressive and Dementia Network has a Permission to Contact system – complementary to *Join Dementia Research* – which also allows you to opt in to find out about research opportunities. Here you can permit researchers to look at your medical records to match you with the most appropriate research studies. They can check if you have any conditions or take any medications that would exclude you from participating, saving time and disappointment compared to finding this out later. The *Global Alzheimer Platform* – another registry of current dementia research – is also a source of research opportunities, particularly in North America.

Will I get any benefit from taking part in research?

Taking part in a trial can sometimes give you access to new treatments. However, there is usually an equal chance that you will receive the inactive placebo rather than the treatment under study. Even if you receive the active treatment, the trial may show that it doesn't work or that there are side effects which outweigh any potential benefit. Similarly, although you might receive travel expenses and possibly some minimal compensation for the time you spend taking part in a trial, this is not a way to get rich!

For most people, the motivation to participate in research is not to gain a direct benefit for themselves but to help people who will come after them. Tom is always impressed by the altruism of his research participants. They want to help future generations access better treatments and know that research is the way to achieve this.

How will research impact me?

There is a lot of evidence that clinical outcomes are better in research-active hospitals compared to ones where research is not taking place. At a personal level, many participants value their regular contact with the research team – often over several years – and benefit from the stimulation and feeling of empowerment.

What are the drawbacks of taking part in research?

Whatever research you choose to take part in, you will need to invest some of your time – mainly travelling to and attending appointments. Should you take part in a clinical trial, you will likely have to attend the hospital for a series of appointments (some of which might last all day), possibly over several years. You might have blood tests and other investigations, such as brain scans.

Again, in a clinical trial, you might experience side effects from the drug treatment. Under normal circumstances, you won't know for sure until the end of the trial whether you were receiving the active treatment or placebo. However, if you become unwell or in the event of any other emergency, you can be 'unblinded' to allow the medical team treating you to know the medication you have been receiving.

Can I take part in research into new treatments?

Yes, you can! Many clinical trials of new drug treatments are looking to recruit people with dementia – particularly in the early stages – and mild cognitive impairment to take part in trials. See above for details of where to look to find out about research opportunities near you.

Treatment means more than medication, though; research studies also investigate other treatments for dementia, such as psychological therapies, music, and different models of care. These kinds of studies should be accessible through the same routes highlighted above.

Can I help researchers without being a research participant?

As mentioned above, researchers have been guilty of doing research *to* people with dementia rather than *with* them. However, many research groups now involve people with lived experience of dementia and interested members of the general public at all stages of their projects. For example, you could help guide research questions or to design a research study from the start. Some research projects are 'co-produced' with people with lived experience of dementia as co-researchers on an equal footing with the 'professional' researchers.

In our experience, this is a fun way to do research and leads to insights and ideas that would never have emerged doing things the traditional way. For instance, Tom was involved in a project speaking with people with dementia who were given a diagnosis remotely – either by phone or video call – during the COVID-19 lockdowns. We worked on this project with a fascinating group of individuals with lived experience of dementia. They co-produced the interview schedules we used to speak with people, read through transcripts of the interviews, identified recurring themes, and produced animated films and a podcast series about the project (*Diagnosing Dementia during COVID-19*).

There can still be an element of tokenism when including people with lived experience in research studies, but their meaningful involvement is, rightly, becoming the norm. It remains much more prevalent in university-based research than in commercial clinical trials.

Can I be a researcher?

Yes! If you are even slightly interested, we encourage you to contact local researchers to find out how you could be involved. As mentioned above, not every researcher involves people with lived experience in their research yet, but enough of us are. We would be very grateful for your valuable contribution.

Our research participants tell us that they enjoy participating in research, and evidence suggests that it does you good. Everyone should give it a go!

10

What are the main stages of dementia?

When does someone merit a diagnosis of dementia?

There is some uncertainty about where to draw the line between dementia and non-dementia. Many factors influence the pencil-and-paper cognitive tests you complete during a memory assessment, including your educational attainment, whether you are completing them in your first language, and whether you have completed similar tests recently (psychologists call this a 'practice effect').

As such, while cut-off points suggest that someone scoring below a particular score might have dementia, this has to be considered in light of their whole presentation. Furthermore, as we see above, other conditions may present with cognitive impairment, so *how* someone completes the cognitive test is also important. A depressed person may score poorly but answer 'I don't know' rather than get the answers wrong.

A person's day-to-day function is even more complex to assess. What an 85-year-old should be able to manage is a value judgement with no set criteria. The clinician will have their ideas, as will the person being assessed and their relatives. Defining when someone is no longer *fully* independent is therefore imprecise. The same person might be classified on one side or the other of the line on different days, depending on who else the doctor had seen that day and, perhaps, what they had for lunch. Also, the level of support a person has around them is very relevant.

1. No impairment 2. Very mild cognitive decline 3. Mild cognitive decline
4. Moderate cognitive decline – mild dementia 5. Moderately severe cognitive decline – moderate dementia   (someone from this stage can no longer live without assistance) 6. Severe cognitive decline – moderately severe dementia 7. Very severe cognitive decline – severe dementia

Figure 10.1 Reisberg's seven stages of dementia (1–3 are pre-dementia; 4–7 are dementia)

One popular classification of the different stages of dementia is Dr Barry Reisberg's seven stages of dementia (see Figure 10.1). Although the dementia/non-dementia line is between stages 3 and 4, there remains an element of judgement about how much difficulty with day-to-day activities is enough to merit a diagnosis of dementia.

What is mild cognitive impairment (MCI)?

Figure 10.2 shows the progression of disease in someone who develops dementia. Mild cognitive impairment (MCI) is a description applied to people with some changes in their memory but no significant difficulties carrying out day-to-day activities. However, what constitutes significant difficulties is a value judgement. For this reason, we believe mild cognitive impairment is a description and not a diagnosis.

Mild cognitive impairment is a high-risk state for dementia, but how high the risk is not always clear. Of those described as having mild cognitive impairment in a memory clinic setting, about one in nine people might develop dementia over the next year, and eight out of nine people will either remain stable or even improve! The important message is that not everyone who has mild cognitive impairment goes on to develop dementia.

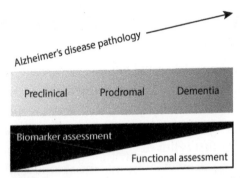

Figure 10.2 The progression through preclinical and prodromal Alzheimer disease to dementia

Over time, Alzheimer disease pathology accumulates through the brain. A person who will eventually develop Alzheimer dementia passes through the stages of preclinical Alzheimer disease and prodromal Alzheimer disease (or mild cognitive impairment). Early on, it will only be possible to identify Alzheimer disease through brain scans or lumbar puncture/spinal tap (biomarkers). As symptoms develop, the importance of functional assessment increases.

Adapted with permission from C. W. Ritchie et al. (2017) The Edinburgh Consensus: preparing for the advent of disease-modifying therapies for Alzheimer's disease. *Alzheimer's Research & Therapy* 9: 85 <https://doi.org/10.1186/s13195-017-0312-4>

How does dementia progress over time?

A simple way to visualize the progress of dementia symptoms is to imagine a set of fairy lights, where each light represents a skill, function, or memory. In a healthy brain, each light is fully lit. As dementia starts, some of those lights begin to flicker. Over time, as the disease progresses, it spreads through the brain, causing more lights to flicker and, eventually, some or all the lights to go out.

Depending on the type of dementia, different symptoms will be more pronounced in the early stages. As the disease becomes more advanced and symptoms accumulate, all types of dementia begin to resemble one another. Although a typical disease progression can be described for each type of dementia, everyone's experience of the disease is unique.

How long will I live after being diagnosed with dementia?

Dementia is a progressive, life-limiting condition, which means that someone diagnosed with any dementia will, on average, live for a shorter time than someone of a similar age without dementia.

There are two main ways in which dementia reduces life expectancy. The first is linked conditions (comorbidities), such as diabetes and cardiovascular disease. The second is the severity of dementia itself in its most advanced stages. A person with late-stage dementia is most likely frail, with a suppressed immune system, will spend more time in bed, and might experience difficulties swallowing. These issues increase the chances of developing additional medical complications, such as infections or cardiovascular problems, that are the immediate 'cause' of death.

The average life expectancy for the main types of dementia are:

- **Alzheimer dementia.** Approximately eight to ten years, generally less if the person is diagnosed in their eighties or nineties. For people diagnosed at a younger age, it is possible, though uncommon, for people to live up to 15–20 years.
- **Vascular dementia.** Approximately five years. This is less than Alzheimer dementia because of the possibility of a stroke or heart attack.
- **Dementia with Lewy bodies.** Approximately six years. Someone with dementia with Lewy bodies is more prone to falls and infections that, again, reduce life expectancy relative to Alzheimer dementia.
- **Frontotemporal dementia.** Approximately six to eight years.

Like any condition, the length of time a person with dementia will live is not predetermined. Good care and support and effective management of a person's general health can help ensure a better quality of life for longer.

Am I going to die of dementia or with dementia?

As is true of any of us, a person with dementia can die of something else (a heart attack, a stroke, cancer, or an accident) at any time. Any of these could be the event which ends the person's life, or they may recover – but often not to the same level they were beforehand.

Someone whose dementia progresses to an advanced stage will become increasingly frail and require greater levels of care. In the last stages of life, they may need to be nursed in bed. As the brain deteriorates, controlling different bodily functions becomes more difficult. The person may become incontinent of urine, faeces or both.

In the later stages, coordinating the muscles required for swallowing can become more difficult, and they may not even be able to swallow saliva. Changing the consistency of food and fluids in consultation with speech and language therapists can help. Still, there is a high risk of food or fluids being aspirated into the lungs (going down 'the wrong way'), possibly resulting in a chest infection, which could be fatal. Indeed, pneumonia is a common cause of death in someone with advanced dementia.

Is it always best to intervene if I become unwell?

This question demonstrates the importance of anticipatory care discussions. Involving someone with advanced dementia in these discussions can present challenges and, in practice, these discussions are often with family members. By this, we mean sensitively discussing 'what if?' scenarios to consider the pros and cons of intervening. Possible scenarios include what if my relative fell and broke a bone, developed pneumonia, or became unwell enough to die?

The benefits of any intervention should be weighed against potential harms. For someone with advanced dementia, the upheaval and possible distress of transfer to another setting is usually one significant factor. Consequently, it can be better to focus on symptom control, comfort, and dignity rather than aggressive treatment. An exception is when a bone is broken. In this event, only an X-ray and appropriate treatment, usually in hospital, are effective.

Should someone develop pneumonia, for example, it might be appropriate to treat this with oral antibiotics if the person can swallow. However, it might not be appropriate to use intravenous antibiotics (through a drip), particularly if this would require transfer somewhere else. Often, it is better to manage symptoms, keep the person comfortable, and ensure they have a dignified death.

A good ending is possible – though not guaranteed – and can help the grieving process for those left behind. A useful resource is the 'Good Life – Good Death – Good Grief' project run by the Scottish Partnership for Palliative Care (<www.goodlifedeath-grief.org.uk/>).

11

What are the common cognitive symptoms of dementia?

Some symptoms are more typical of early dementia or more advanced illness, but there are no hard-and-fast rules. People might experience symptoms typical of a later stage earlier, and vice versa. However, throughout the illness, symptoms may improve or disappear completely, while others may emerge.

Why do I forget things and repeat myself?

Short-term memory loss is the symptom most people associate with dementia and is often the reason they contact their doctor. Difficulty recalling phone numbers or appointments or whether you have eaten can make everyday life a challenge. It can leave you feeling confused, disoriented and anxious.

Long-term memories are better preserved and can come to the surface when short-term memories are less accessible. Long-term memories are a collection of sights, sounds and smells stored in the brain. Listening to a song played at your wedding or looking at a family holiday photograph could transport you back to that time. Many people with dementia can recount memories from their younger life in detail. For this reason, they can mix up the past and the present, thinking they are at a different stage in life.

If your memory is not as good as it once was, you might become more reliant on others. The text box below outlines some suggestions on how you and your carers can adapt to and cope with changes in your memory.

- **Write short instructions.** Even simple tasks like making a cup of tea comprise many steps: locating the kitchen, knowing what you need and in which order, finding the right components, then using each of them correctly. Write short instructions for any multi-step tasks and leave what you need visible.
- **Set reminders.** Write reminders of upcoming events, appointments, and one-off tasks on a whiteboard. Limit the information to one day at a time to reduce the potential for confusion or anxiety. Display signs in appropriate places to remind you to take your keys, lock the door when going out, and do other regular tasks. Use assistive technology – mobile phones, tablets, and virtual assistants – to set reminders to take medication, eat regularly, and attend appointments.
- **Keep things in one place.** Get into the habit of keeping the items you use regularly, such as keys, phone, glasses, and your wallet or purse, in one visible place.
- **Keep a diary.** Memories of even recent events and conversations can be difficult to recall. Record what you can remember in the form of a diary or log.

For your carer

As a carer, you may find the following suggestions helpful:

- **Repeat or write down answers.** If a person with dementia asks repeated questions, avoid letting them know you have already told them. If they are asking, it's because they genuinely can't remember. Asking can also reflect their underlying confusion and anxiety. Instead, offer simple, easy-to-understand answers that you can repeat and offer reassurance as appropriate.
- **A short pencil is better than a long memory.** You could also write down the answer so that the person can find information without needing to ask again.
- **Allow time, and use prompts.** Any extra pressure or stress can worsen the problem if the person cannot find the word they want to use. Allow them time to finish what they want to say. If you don't fully understand what they want to say, try to make sense of the context. Use prompts and cues – such as showing the person pictures or objects or describing the context – to help them

understand you. For example, if you have a visitor but the person with dementia has forgotten who they are, use the visitor's name and subtly explain why they are there.

- **Reassure the person that they are safe.** If a person with dementia is unsettled at home, they might be 'time-shifting' and recalling a past home or place of security. As a carer, listen to their concerns, reassure them that they are safe, and try to work out what they are feeling. It can help to talk about their former home and what it means to them. Doing so might help identify what they need to feel settled and secure. If the 'home' they are referring to does not exist, it could be that they are feeling generally confused, anxious and insecure. Display familiar items and photographs of familiar people, and retain the familiar layout of their home environment to help them feel 'at home'.
- **Compile a photo album.** As dementia progresses, even the most familiar faces, including the person's own – their reflection or in photographs – might become unrecognizable. They could feel you have strangers or intruders in your home. They might not recognize a person because they no longer look like the person they see in their long-term memory. A wife or husband aged 80 years will not wholly resemble the bride or groom aged 20.
- **Try to remain calm.** Your response will either heighten the person's distress or help them feel more at ease. The sound of your voice, offering reassurance, can help reorient a person. Compile a photo album to display, in chronological order, memorable episodes from your life together. Doing so can help the person join the dots between present and past. Wear clothes or apply perfume or aftershave to trigger memories and help the person recognize you.

Why do I keep getting lost?

You might still have a strong sense of where you want to go – a shop, favourite café, or the hairdresser – but be less sure how to get there. Over time, even familiar routes can become more challenging to navigate. Any diversion or distraction as you travel could complicate your journey further.

Very often, a person with dementia will have a clear purpose in mind when what is sometimes (slightly insultingly) described as 'wandering'. We try to say 'walking with purpose', which suggests there is a reason you walk, such as continuing an existing habit, counteracting boredom, using up energy or relieving pain. You might not always be able to explain your reasons for going out or you could forget. Carers should note any pattern to your behaviour, such as going out at the same time that you used to walk the dog, and help you to remain independent and safe. They could walk with you or use appropriate assistive technology, such as a GPS device. Many devices feature 'geofencing' (an alert that triggers if you go beyond a set boundary), two-way calling, and an SOS button. Your family and carers can quickly locate you using a Smartphone or computer, helping you remain independent while providing a safety net and peace of mind for them.

Carrying a form of ID and alerting others in the community can be another layer of security. A simple card showing your name, medical details, and emergency contact is sufficient. Your carer, another family member, or voluntary or paid support might accompany you if you cannot find your way when out alone. You or your carer might let others in the local community know that you have dementia and could get lost. In Scotland, the *Purple Alert* smartphone app (<www.alzscot.org/purple-alert>) alerts people locally when someone with dementia goes missing; equivalent systems may be available elsewhere. The Herbert Protocol (<www.scotland.police.uk/what-s-happening/missing-persons/the-herbert-protocol/>) helps the police and other agencies collaborate in such situations.

As the disease progresses, the risks associated with going out alone can be significant. Even with GPS, going out alone could expose you to practical dangers, like traffic, other people, hypothermia or dehydration, and emotional distress. Such risks are unlikely to deter you from 'walking with purpose'. You might leave home without your family or carers realizing, sometimes taking your GPS device, sometimes not. In such cases, where safety is paramount, your carer might fit door sensors to alert them when you attempt to leave.

You should still be supported to walk regularly. If not, you could feel trapped and frustrated. If your actual 'need' is not to walk but to use the toilet or find something to eat, then carers can help you feel settled by supporting you to meet your needs. You could put signs up at home to help you find your way and camouflage exits. Stimulating activity can also reduce the chances of you becoming disoriented.

Why do I struggle to plan, solve problems, and make decisions?

Most activities – from cooking a meal to making a journey – require foresight, planning, and an ability to deal with the unexpected. As your dementia progresses, you might find that completing routine tasks independently and safely is affected by changes in concentration and difficulties following multiple steps, understanding new ideas, or solving problems.

Can I still make decisions after being diagnosed with dementia?

Dementia can affect your ability to make some decisions, but a diagnosis of dementia does not mean that you cannot make any decisions. Your judgement may change with dementia, and this can often precede memory loss as the first noticeable symptom. If your judgement is impaired, you might find it harder to weigh up the various factors necessary to make a decision. You might not be able to evaluate and predict the potential outcomes and consequences of the decisions you make. Impaired judgement can affect your health and safety, financial situation, social relationships, personal appearance, and driving.

'Mental capacity' is the legal term for whether or not you can make a specific decision. A diagnosis of dementia does not automatically mean that you now lack capacity. Indeed, capacity is not all or nothing but depends on the type of decision. Even if you lack capacity to make some decisions, you will be able to make other decisions for yourself.

This may become an issue when a big decision needs to be made. For example, you might need to decide whether to move into care or receive medical treatments.

In Scotland, you are held to lack legal capacity if you are incapable of at least one of acting, making, communicating, understanding, or retaining the memory of decisions. The onus is not on you to prove your decision-making capacity, but your doctor might speak with you to clarify if you have capacity to make a specific decision.

In general, you should be supported to make your own decisions for as long as possible, and always be involved in everyday decisions – for example, what to eat and wear and how to spend your time. You might find it helpful to be offered a narrower range of choices or be shown objects or pictures to make choices easier to understand. In doing so, people around you can support you to be independent and feel in control. This can reduce some of the frustration you might experience if you feel you are not being listened to and that some decisions are being made on your behalf.

Why do I sometimes feel literally lost for words?

Dysphasia means that a person has difficulty with their language or speech. Dysphasia in dementia can mean you are more hesitant in your speech, taking longer to find the right word before speaking. Sometimes you might use the incorrect word, often starting with the same letter as the word you are looking for, or you might describe what the word means. You can know what you want to say – the words are on the 'tip of your tongue' – but cannot say it. Your understanding of what is being said can often be better than your ability to speak, especially in the early stages of dementia. With dysphasia, your ability to write can also diminish.

Not finding the right word repeatedly might cause you to feel embarrassed and frustrated. As this become more noticeable, you might feel like withdrawing from situations where you will be asked questions or expected to follow a conversation and join in. The problem might be magnified in a busy environment – multiple conversations at once, background noise like the television, or lots of visual distractions.

If you experience dysphasia, a speech and language therapist may be able to help you retain your communication skills for longer. The text box outlines some strategies that a speech and language therapist might suggest.

- **Be patient.** Give yourself extra time when speaking. The more pressure you place on yourself to find the right word, the harder it will be. Try not to blame yourself or feel embarrassed if you cannot find the right word straight away.
- **Describe.** Describe what the thing looks like or what it is for. These clues can help the person you are interacting with determine what you are referring to.
- **Associate.** Refer to something related to what you want to talk about. It might prompt the right words to follow or sufficiently convey the meaning you intended.
- **Use synonyms.** Use a word that means the same or something similar.
- **The first letter.** Go through the alphabet. When you get to the first letter of the word you are looking for, it might help you to say it.
- **Act it out.** Act out the word you are looking for with your hands or body. If you can't act it out, moving your hands or tapping on a surface can sometimes bring the word to mind.

- **Draw it.** Keep a pen and paper to hand to sketch what it is you can't find the words for.
- **Look it up.** Sometimes the word you are looking for will be written down or be pictured somewhere – in a newspaper, magazine, book, or on your phone.
- **Narrow it down.** Tell the person you are interacting with the general topic. This might tell them whether you are talking about a person, place, or thing.
- **Come back later.** Reduce the pressure on yourself to find the right word right away. The word you were looking for will sometimes come to you when you are busy with something else.

When speaking and being understood, the words we use are often the least significant part of communication. The non-verbal aspects of communication – tone of voice, eye contact, and body language – can carry greater weight.

For people with dementia, non-verbal communication can be even more important. It might take longer to make sense of what your ears hear and to respond how you would like. How the people you interact with speak and their body language will affect how well you understand and respond.

For your carer: tips for communication
- Use words with fewer syllables.
- Present only one or two pieces of information at a time.
- Take more time over what you are saying.
- Pause to allow the person to engage with what you are saying.
- Use a soft and gentle tone of voice.
- Maintain eye contact.
- Keep body language open and relaxed.

As with most dementia symptoms, the degree to which word-finding difficulties affect you will vary day-to-day and depend on other factors, such as tiredness, dehydration, or pain. A quiet, calm environment is also likely to help good, effective communication.

Your carers (and other people) can help you understand and participate in the conversation by using what they know about you and their observations to decide the best way to communicate. For example, they might use visual cues to help make it easier to understand what a word refers to. Asking you to put your shoes on to get ready to go out might seem sensible until you return with the laundry basket. Instead, pointing at or holding the shoes while asking will help you take the right action and remove the embarrassment or frustration you might feel at making a mistake. Likewise, carers could show you a few options – about what to eat, for example – to help you make a choice and feel more in control, empowered, and valued.

Why do I get confused about time?

Being disoriented in time is called 'time-shifting'. Time-shifting can be distressing, especially if the people around you do not understand why it is happening. Suppose you are confused and feel like you are in a different time, potentially decades earlier in your life. In that case, you might notice significant differences from the actual present. For example, you might understand your deceased parents to be still alive. Similarly, the house where you live now might not be the home where you expect to be.

Short-term memory difficulties mean that memories from your past can play a new and confusing role in understanding and making sense of the present. They can also be dangerous. For example, making a cup of tea in a modern kitchen could be risky as the electric kettle does not work the same way as a whistling kettle.

In the earlier and middle stages of dementia, time-shifting is likely to be short-lived, coming and going across a day, particularly if you are tired, dehydrated, hungry, in pain, or developing an infection.

In this respect, time-shifting has a lot in common with delusions. Both the immediate experience and how your carers can effectively respond to reduce the potential for distress are similar. We say 'potential for distress' because time-shifting episodes are not always upsetting. Some people are content essentially reliving happy memories. However, not all memories are happy, and even the happiest might be distressing when contrasted with present realities.

When you are time-shifting, your carer's understanding of reality will differ from yours. As with delusions, it might help if your carer can 'enter into' your reality, confirming rather than contradicting your sense of things. It can also help if your carers remain positive and relaxed and listen carefully to you to work out the memories you might be responding to. If you are upset, they should acknowledge this and help you feel heard, not dismiss or ignore your question or concerns. The text box explores a common example.

For your carer

Let's look at a common example of time-shifting and some ways in which you as a carer could respond. Should a person with dementia ask to see a relative who is now deceased, you might sensitively remind them of the fact. However, this might upset them because it could feel like they are learning this for the first time. Moreover, they might forget the answer and ask the same question again hours or even minutes later. You could either repeat the honest response and replay the emotional distress or offer a potentially more consoling 'untruth'.

Alternatively, you could answer the question indirectly, tapping into the feelings behind it. You could ask if the person misses their relative and make time to reminisce, potentially using photographs to help reorient the person to the present. In this way, you might also understand if there are any unmet needs underlying the person's question. For example, they might miss the security and comfort once provided by the deceased parent. By reflecting on the importance of the deceased – 'You must really miss them' – you might give similar comfort.

You might not always have the time or energy to respond with as much empathy. Instead, you might tell the person with dementia that their relative is at work or on holiday and will be back 'later' or 'in a few weeks'. By gesturing towards a future that will never arrive, you are anticipating that the person will, if not forget, then at least temporarily move on from the issue.

You might find this approach uncomfortable because it is a form of deception. If the person with dementia realizes, they might become more suspicious. You might feel like you are taking advantage of the cognitive changes the person is experiencing.

Given that every person, relationship, and scenario is unique, there is no absolute right or wrong answer. In our experience, though, carers who use the above-mentioned approaches help limit the amount of unnecessary emotional distress for both.

Finally, the 'right' response one time might be the 'wrong' response next time. However, as much as possible, consistency when answering the same question is helpful, rather than shifting between truth, half-truth, and untruth.

12

What are the common behavioural and psychological symptoms of dementia?

Why might I behave inappropriately?

The word 'disinhibition' describes behaviours that break social norms and are out of character for the person. Examples include making inappropriate remarks, swearing, undressing, or touching oneself (or others) in public. Family members often find these symptoms upsetting.

People with frontotemporal dementia are more likely to display disinhibited behaviours than those living with other types of dementia. The frontal lobes of the brain act as a 'filter' for what is appropriate behaviour.

You might not recognize the social norm you have transgressed, so if you act 'inappropriately', it is unlikely to be deliberate. How other people respond to your behaviour might make you feel confused, distressed, or embarrassed.

For your carer

For carers, it is helpful to understand the possible reasons why someone might behave in a particular way and to support them in addressing the issue. For example, we might all remove a layer of clothing if we are too hot to try to cool down. However, the person with dementia might no longer recognize the taboo on public nakedness and remove more clothing than other people would.

Being mindful of the person's mood, unmet needs, and environmental factors can make it less likely that they will behave inappropriately. By contrast, telling the person off during or after the fact is unlikely to prevent the behaviour happening again and could make them feel ashamed.

Why don't I feel like doing anything?

Apathy – a profound decrease in motivation – affects up to two-thirds of people living with dementia. It is most common in frontotemporal dementia, dementia with Lewy bodies, and Parkinson disease dementia. The physiological cause of apathy is damage to the brain's frontal lobes, responsible for motivation, planning, and sequencing.

If you experience apathy, you might withdraw from everyday activities. You might no longer work on hobbies, follow your interests, or attend social engagements. You could neglect necessary activities such as housework and gardening. Withdrawing can start a vicious cycle: by no longer engaging, you might lose confidence and skills more quickly and become more apathetic.

People with dementia experiencing apathy have a lower quality of life. Their emotional state also affects family and carers who need extra energy and buoyancy to encourage them to complete tasks and practise basic self-care.

Depression is often confused with apathy, though the similarity is only superficial. Depression usually means the person with dementia feels sad or 'fed up', hopeless, and guilty. They may no longer get pleasure from activities they previously enjoyed. By contrast, if you are apathetic, you can appear unconcerned by your symptoms or current life experience but can still enjoy things when you get involved. Cholinesterase inhibitor medication can alleviate a degree of apathy and boost motivation, memory, and concentration. Antidepressants are unlikely to be helpful.

Music, art, reminiscence, and cognitive stimulation sessions could motivate you to remain engaged and improve your mental health. Following a daily routine can provide structure and security, help you feel you are accomplishing things, and maintain your confidence and skills. Doing so could put the vicious cycle in reverse.

If your carers adopt a positive approach focused on your strengths and skills rather than what you can't do, you will have an improved quality of life. They must avoid the misperception that you are simply being lazy.

Why do I feel so depressed?

As many as two in five people with dementia also experience depression. Low mood, anxiety, agitation, and delusions (false beliefs) are all possible signs of dementia-related depression.

If you feel this way, you should talk to your GP. Depression is a treatable condition, and antidepressant medication and talking therapies can help. If depressive symptoms are alleviated, you might find the 'ordinary' challenges of living with dementia easier to cope with.

Carers, family, and friends can help by creating positive routines (made up of activities meaningful to you) and encouraging you to continue to be socially and physically active.

Why do I always feel anxious?

As your memory changes, retaining new information and recalling familiar places and people becomes more challenging. As a result, you might feel chronically uncertain, insecure, and anxious. You might feel restless, pace, struggle to sleep, and cling to significant objects. You might find it difficult to settle in the company of others and seek out your carer around the house. Your carer might become your point of security and certainty in an overwhelming world.

For your carer

Carers in this situation should offer reassurance and empathy. Remind the person that you love and care for them. Show that you understand and empathize with their experience of living with dementia. Make clear that they are not alone and that you will continue to be there for them.

When reassuring a person, always approach from the front, where they can see you. Use simple statements, such as 'I'm here, I will help you'. For some people, depending on their need for physical space at the point when they are distressed, physical touch – on their arm, for example – can offer a calming, non-verbal confirmation of your presence. It is important to respect what the person with dementia feels, however minor the issue that is upsetting them might seem to you. Statements such as 'It sounds like you are upset that...' or 'I see that you're feeling sad about...' directly address the emotion and underlying cause. It can then be helpful to either offer to help resolve the issue (i.e., finding a lost item) or, if appropriate, a diversion: 'Let's get something to eat first, then we'll get everything sorted out.'

For some carers, it will be possible to leave notes as a reminder of where they have gone and when they will return. However, you might consider arranging support if the person can no longer read, doesn't remember to look at notes, or is not safe to be left alone. A paid or voluntary companion can develop a meaningful relationship with the person you care for, engage them in activities, and enable you to take a regular break.

Some medications can be prescribed to reduce anxiety and help the person with dementia feel more emotionally stable.

Why does how I feel change so often?

Your mood and emotional state can change frequently when you have dementia and often without obvious cause. You might be responding to changes in your abilities or potentially feeling scared, confused, or tired. You might also be in pain, uncomfortable, too hot or cold, need to use the toilet, or feel bored and under-stimulated.

Mood swings can also be the by-product of untreated psychiatric disorders, diet, caffeine, or overstimulation from too much activity, feeling rushed, and excess clutter and noise. You might be less able to describe how you are feeling. Instead, you might express yourself by crying or an angry outburst.

Even when the disease is more advanced, you will continue to experience a range of positive emotions, such as joy and love.

Routines can enhance your quality of life and help reduce the chances of mood and behavioural changes. You and your carer will come to know when negative mood swings occur and can use diversions, such as playing music or going for a walk.

For your carer

As a carer, put yourself in the place of the person with dementia to help identify which 'unmet needs' they might be responding to and offer the best response. Although it can be challenging when you feel tired and stressed, try to keep the perspective that mood swings are a normal part of dementia, not the person deliberately making life more difficult.

Why do I sometimes think and feel things that are untrue?

Many people with dementia experience delusions (false beliefs) that affect their perception of reality, including the nature of their relationships with others. With little cause or evidence, a person might conclude they are being watched, that someone is stealing their belongings, or that a loved one is unfaithful. A family member or friend might be a stranger; something you have stored away might be stolen. Your ability to logically think through a situation is affected.

For your carer

As a carer, you will find delusions difficult to disprove. They feel as real to the person with dementia as the reality of you reading this sentence. If someone told you that you are, in fact, not reading this sentence, you would likely feel affronted. A person with dementia might take this further, potentially becoming verbally or physically aggressive because of changes in the way they think.

Rather than correct the person's sense of reality, try to empathize with what they are experiencing. Acknowledge their emotional distress and help redress the situation – for example, by offering to find a 'stolen' object. When speaking, think about your tone of voice. Although you might feel stressed and frustrated, try to remain calm and reassuring. Engaging the person in meaningful, enjoyable activities can divert their attention from the delusion so they forget it. At other times it might be necessary to go along with the delusion until they move on to a different topic and feel calmer. If attempts to help fail or seem to intensify the person's distress, it's OK to leave the room to collect your thoughts. This approach can sometimes 'reset' the person's mood. On your return, positively and confidently present a new scenario, such as making a cup of tea or going for a walk.

It can help to keep important items in a safe place and to hold spares of things that are most likely to be misplaced. Changes in sight and hearing can increase confusion, so you should arrange regular eye and hearing tests. Eating and drinking reduce the risk of fatigue and confusion while adhering to a routine can help a person feel safe and secure. By keeping the layout of the person's home environment the same, they will feel more oriented in space. Displaying photographs of family and friends at different stages of their life can help the person recognize them in the present. Sometimes, if delusions are persistent and cause distress, a doctor may suggest medication (an antipsychotic) to treat them.

Should delusions appear suddenly, contact their doctor to work out if the person is experiencing delirium. Delirium can be triggered by an underlying, potentially treatable physical cause, such as an infection.

Always listen carefully to the person with dementia. Do not dismiss their every worry as a sign of a delusional state. Not only are their concerns real to them, but people with dementia can be more vulnerable. It is possible that they are being taken advantage of in some way.

Does everyone with dementia become aggressive?

One persistent, prejudicial view of dementia is that everyone who develops the disease will become angry and aggressive. In reality, such behaviours are often triggered by something specific. As such, it is not only people who were previously hot-tempered who behave aggressively. Previously mild-mannered people might also be prone to angry outbursts.

Aggression takes two forms: verbal and physical. Verbal aggression can start as a raised voice and objection but can become shouting, screaming, and direct threats. Physical aggression includes anything that causes – or could cause – physical harm to another person or thing.

Aggression in dementia can have many causes. It can be the result of the brain changes of dementia. Medications can sometimes induce side effects, including agitation and aggression. Aggression can stem from hunger, thirst, or pain. Delusions and hallucinations can also cause the person to react aggressively, often in self-defence against a perceived threat.

Sometimes aggression may reflect poor relations with the people around them. We are all likely to react negatively to these experiences. However, a person with dementia might be less able to make sense of the situation and moderate their response accordingly, resulting in more extreme displays of anger and aggression.

A person with dementia will likely experience varying degrees of fear and uncertainty brought about by memory loss, confusion, and disorientation. These symptoms can cause them to misinterpret the intentions of those around them and react defensively. As such, carers need to be aware of how they communicate. You might consider simplifying what you say, how much you say, and at what speed, as well as your body language and facial expressions.

Many people with dementia feel frustrated because of their changing abilities or because their carers – with the best intentions – take over. Many carers do this because it is difficult to see someone struggle or because it is quicker to do it themselves. But frustration can sometimes spill over into aggression.

Many people with dementia become more isolated. Reasons for this include apathy, loss of confidence, changes in communication skills, and deteriorating physical health. As a result, they can feel lonely, bored, and under-stimulated, which can lead to aggression. Even those who are active socially can, as their memory loss worsens, forget that they have been busy earlier in the day.

Why do I feel worse later in the day?

'Sundowning' is something that affects one in five people living with dementia. Mood and behaviours change as the afternoon turns into the evening. You might feel restless, confused, and irritable, and may even experience hallucinations. Sometimes this will last for many hours and might disrupt your sleep.

Sundowning is not fully understood but potential triggers include:

- dementia-related changes to your 'body clock'
- discomfort resulting from hunger or pain
- boredom
- fear and anxiety produced by shadows
- reduced sensory stimulation as daylight fades
- less need for sleep (an average of five and a half hours as we get older).

For many people with dementia, sundowning can mean they stop recognizing their home and sometimes their family.

For your carer

As a carer, listen carefully to the person's feelings, offer reassurance, and suggest positive diversions to help the person be more settled.

As with any behaviour, it is usually possible to identify a pattern to sundowning, such as the time of afternoon/evening it occurs and potential triggers. It might then be possible to adapt your routines to prevent or reduce the impact on the person and you.

You can support the person with dementia to be socially active and participate in appropriate exercise daily. But remember, too much activity can be overstimulating and tiring.

For some people, a short early afternoon rest can help and might prevent you from napping later. An early nap can also help you sleep longer and better overnight.

After exposing the person to lots of natural light during the day, closing the curtains and switching on soft artificial lighting can mark the transition into an evening routine. Try to avoid potentially stressful activities like bathing or showering around this time. Minimize triggers such as excess noise, bright lights, caffeine, and alcohol, which can add to the person's confusion and restlessness. By contrast, meaningful therapeutic activities, including listening to familiar music, reading aloud, massage, or spending time with pets, can help the person feel more relaxed.

Alongside adopting some or all of the strategies above, a GP may be able to help. Pain, illness, a sleep disorder, or medication side effects can all contribute to the problem.

13

What are the common sensory symptoms of dementia?

Sensory symptoms are changes in sight, hearing, smell, taste, and touch. Sensation is a difficult thing to describe, even in the absence of dementia. These symptoms can be difficult for anyone else to grasp fully, however well described they are.

Sensory loss can further complicate a person's experience of the sensory symptoms associated with dementia. Glasses and hearing aids can improve deteriorating eyesight and hearing, but some people with dementia find them challenging to use.

Why do I see things differently now?

Changes in the visual parts of the brain can make it harder to know exactly what your eyes see. This can result in visual misperceptions or illusions. You might also misidentify faces and objects or struggle to judge distances. Some misperceptions are embarrassing or frightening. Others make everyday spaces more challenging to move around safely.

Common examples of misperceptions are:

- black mats that look like holes
- swirls on a carpet appearing as snakes
- patterns of fruit on a tablecloth looking three-dimensional, causing a person to reach out as if to pick a fruit up
- a change in flooring seeming like a step.

Visual misperceptions can increase your risk of falling as steps and pavement edges can appear larger or smaller than they really are.

Likewise, the distance between you and the seat you are preparing to sit on might be greater than expected. If your eyes see a vehicle moving towards you, but your brain thinks it is farther away than it actually is, you might walk into the road in front of it.

Eyesight naturally changes as we age, and you may develop conditions such as macular degeneration and glaucoma. It is important to have regular check-ups with an optician, wear the correct glasses, and ensure they are clean.

Home adaptations can help you safely move around – for example, by ensuring bright, even lighting to reduce shadows; creating colour contrasts to make it easier to identify objects and gauge distances; or fitting plain carpets. As your vision changes, you might increasingly rely on memories and habits to move around your home. Try to keep the physical layout of rooms more or less as they were.

When outside, carrying a white stick can help you 'feel' environments and reduce your dependence on visual perception. A stick also signals to others that you might need extra consideration. Wherever you are, take your time to make sure you move around safely.

If you find your local area difficult to move around, tell the person responsible, for example, the café manager or a local councillor. If it affects you, other people living with dementia will likely be affected. Indeed, environmental adaptations made to help people with dementia might improve everyone's experience.

For your carer

As a carer, try not to point out the mistakes that might follow from visual misperceptions, such as wrongly identifying a person or picking up an object other than the one needed. This could knock the person's confidence. Instead, you could ask visitors to introduce themselves on arrival, offer reminders during the conversation, and make it known when they leave or re-enter the room. When handing a person an object, describe what it is for and how to use it. Offer reassurance to the person to help them feel safe, for example, if the floor is blue, which might be perceived as water.

How does hearing affect my experience of dementia?

Hearing loss is now seen as an important risk factor for dementia. Mild hearing loss might double the chance of developing dementia. Moderate hearing loss, meanwhile, pushes the risk to three to four times as likely.

If you have dementia, a hearing impairment can complicate your experience of the illness. First, you might be unable to communicate the problems associated with hearing loss. Your frustration at this might be wrongly attributed to dementia when they are primarily hearing related.

Second, even without hearing loss, you might not be able to communicate as well. Hearing loss can worsen language processing and understanding. This can affect your confidence and cause you to withdraw from social activities. You are then at greater risk of isolation, loneliness, and under-stimulation, which, in turn, might lead to anger and aggression.

As with eyesight, you should have regular hearing checks. However, diagnosing and managing hearing loss in a person with dementia is not always straightforward. Both understanding instructions and sharing information might be more difficult. Some audiology departments have specialists qualified to assess you.

Hearing aids can help. They amplify and deliver noise to the ear canal. However, they must be cleaned and maintained and have their batteries replaced as required (once a week for the average hearing aid). Also, ear wax not only dims hearing in the first place but limits the effectiveness of hearing aids. Most hearing aids amplify all sounds, so some people find them unhelpful or uncomfortable in busy environments with background noise.

For some people with dementia, using and looking after their hearing aids is a challenge that requires ongoing support from unpaid or paid carers. Remembering that hearing is an issue, that hearing aids have been prescribed, and how to operate them correctly are all common difficulties.

Regardless of the severity of hearing loss or whether you use hearing aids, additional equipment can help improve your experience and reduce risks. Vibrating alarm clocks, amplified telephones, doorbells, and smoke alarms that flash are some options available. Reducing ambient noise, using soft furnishings, and ensuring good lighting, especially if you lipread, can all lead to better communication.

The other main hearing-related issue some people with dementia experience is hypersensitivity to noise. You might become anxious or distressed in environments with several competing sounds, such as supermarkets or hospitals. To reduce the likelihood of feeling overloaded, try going to shops or cafés at quieter times, reduce background noise at home (such as the television or radio), and relax quietly after being in a busy place.

How does dementia affect my sense of smell and taste?

Smell is our primitive means of detecting danger. Without it, in the modern world, we might not notice a gas leak or that food has gone bad. You might also be less aware of poor hygiene that might prompt you to wash and change your clothes.

Our sense of smell is also integral to what we taste. The tongue alone is a relatively crude measure of taste, sensing only sweet, salty, sour, bitter, and spicy. Because our taste buds are connected to nerves in our brain, they too are affected by dementia. You might start to experience flavour differently, perhaps enjoying some flavours you could not stand before and vice versa. As a result, it is common for people with dementia to note that their appetite is changing.

How does dementia affect what I eat and drink?

People with dementia often develop a 'sweet tooth'. This can be a problem, especially if you are already overweight or at risk of becoming so, with all the health problems that can bring about. You might also have or develop diabetes. Sweet foods are also generally insubstantial and lack nutritional value.

Continue to eat a healthy, balanced diet. You will have more energy, maintain muscle mass and strength, sleep better, and reduce the likelihood of distressed behaviours. Adapting savoury food to incorporate honey or sugar can make a 'proper' meal more appetising, as can herbs and spices or condiments. Substitute fruit or naturally sweet vegetables for biscuits and sweets. If needed, syrup, jam, or honey can increase the sweetness of puddings.

For your carer

As a carer, it won't always be possible to stick to old routines and expectations around food and mealtimes. It is nearly always better for the person to eat – even if what they eat and when is not regular – than to be undernourished. Generally, people with dementia are more at risk of losing than gaining weight, and food becomes less appealing and more difficult to eat. They might not always realize they are hungry and might not recognize food. In the more advanced stages of the disease, the process of chewing and swallowing can be affected. However, food might be one of the last available forms of enjoyment, particularly towards the end of life.

You might find finger foods easier to handle and grazing a variety of foods more appealing than a set meal. Using crockery that contrasts with the food can help, increasing the chance you will eat. Eating without background distractions – television off, an uncluttered table, a plain tablecloth – can help you concentrate on your food. As a carer, creating a mealtime ritual can encourage a person to stay seated. People who eat alone are more likely to stop eating as healthily or as regularly sooner than those who dine with others. Allow the person time to eat, encouraging them to be independent while being mindful of hot food turning cold and unappealing.

Poorly fitting dentures, medications that reduce appetite, and decreased physical activity might also affect your appetite and eating habits.

How does dementia affect my experience of touch?

Touch is integral to the human experience. In the absence of other conditions – such as diabetes – changes in the sensation of touch are uncommon in dementia. The importance of touch remains throughout the illness, however. Even in advanced dementia, holding a hand or receiving a hand massage can be a way to stay connected with others when conversation is no longer possible.

14

What other symptoms might a person with dementia experience?

Will dementia stop me from chewing and swallowing?

People with advanced stage dementia might forget to chew and can also experience physical difficulty chewing and swallowing. Cutting up food and providing smaller portions of softer foods can help, as can input from a speech and language therapist. However, there might still come a time when independent feeding is not safe. In this case, feeding the person and asking a qualified medical professional about appropriate liquid food supplements is advisable.

Will I become incontinent?

Incontinence is most likely to affect people with advanced dementia. By this stage, the disease itself might have caused direct damage to the nerve pathways involved in bladder and bowel control. Both the bladder and bowel are also prone to issues independent of dementia, such as cystitis, weakened pelvic floor muscles, enlarged prostate, and irritable bowel syndrome (IBS). Furthermore, people with advanced dementia are likely to experience reduced mobility, struggle to locate the toilet or communicate their need to go to others, and take longer or else be unable to remove clothes. Finally, incontinence can arise as a side effect of some medications.

Making an appointment with a doctor is the first step when incontinence develops. There are also some practical changes you can make at home. These could include: ensuring the toilet is easy to find (using signs, door labels, and appropriate illumination to help with direction); a raised toilet seat and handrails; the person with dementia wearing clothes that go on and off with minimal effort; and removing things like waste baskets from the bathroom that could be mistaken for a toilet.

It can help to regularly but sensitively ask the person with dementia if they need to use the toilet. A good amount of fruit and vegetables in their diet can reduce the risk of constipation, as can staying hydrated. Avoiding stimulants like caffeine and spicy foods can help prevent faecal incontinence.

Incontinence pads and pants, rubber bedsheets, and commodes are all practical aids that can make the experience of incontinence easier to manage. When out in the community it is good to know where the nearest toilets are. Depending on where you live, there should be schemes such as the UK's 'RADAR key' that can be purchased for a nominal fee to unlock disabled facilities. This scheme also provides an app that maps the whereabouts of all applicable toilets.

Does dementia increase my risk of falling?

Falls are a significant hazard for people with dementia, leading to potential fractures and head injuries, and can even be fatal. Falls are a common reason for hospital admission.

People with dementia are more likely to fall because of their visual perception (potentially misjudging width, depth, and distance), changes in how they walk, and reduced awareness of potential hazards. For example, you are more likely to fall if you are distressed, uncomfortable, in pain, or rushing to use the toilet. Other conditions such as arthritis, infections, visual impairments, heart conditions, and diabetes might make you more confused and less steady on your feet. Side effects from prescribed medications and alcohol intake can also increase your risk.

Totally preventing you from falling is impossible, but the risk can be reduced. A doctor should review your medication and, if you have fallen, should check for injury and identify any underlying cause. Remain as physically active as possible to limit muscle wasting and maintain fitness. A physiotherapist can enhance your mobility and independence, perhaps by exercise (such as seated activity sessions or strength and balance exercises) or by suggesting appropriate walking aids. An occupational therapist can help maximize your independence in daily activities. They might make practical suggestions such as keeping your home environment clear of trip hazards and installing grab rails and bed guards. Depending on where you live, there might be schemes for installing an alarm system. Such systems trigger automatically following a fall, connecting you to a helpline that can alert your family and the emergency services.

15

Advanced dementia

What are the symptoms associated with the later stages of dementia?

Dementia is a progressive illness. Over time, a person's short-term memory difficulties will worsen, but their longer-term memories might remain relatively intact. They will increasingly struggle with other cognitive skills like concentration, planning, and orientation. As a result, they will be less able to complete day-to-day activities and need more support with shopping, cooking, housework, and managing household finances. Eventually, getting washed and dressed becomes more challenging, too, and they will require assistance.

Later on, a person with dementia may become incontinent (of urine, faeces, or both) and might need help to get cleaned up afterwards. Friends and family often provide care in the early stages of dementia. However, it might reach the stage when professional care is necessary.

Over time, symptoms referred to as either 'stress and distress' or 'behavioural and psychological symptoms of dementia' (sometimes abbreviated to BPSD) emerge. They include agitation, aggression, anxiety, apathy, changes in appetite, disinhibition, depression, elation, irritability, mood swings, night-time disturbance, and sometimes psychotic symptoms (delusions or hallucinations). These symptoms can be complex and require tailored treatments, often described as 'person-centred'.

Will I have to move to a care or nursing home when my dementia is advanced?

There usually comes a stage when people with dementia can't live safely without support. Many have family and friends who rally around to provide additional help. However, sometimes people need more care than their families can provide. Alternatively, if a family member who provides most or all support falls ill, outside help might become necessary.

For your carer

Families often have mixed responses to this change; they can feel they should be the ones caring for their relatives. However, it is important to be pragmatic, recognize your limits, acknowledge how caring affects your health and wellbeing, and, if necessary, accept help.

Many people receive care at home, often via their local authority or arranged privately. It can usually involve up to four daily visits to help with specific tasks, including personal care, medication prompts or supervision, and meal preparation. In addition to this care, some families arrange for private cleaners, gardeners, or befrienders.

Should the person require more support during the day, attention overnight, or if their safety is at risk, they might need to move to a home providing residential care. Paying for a comprehensive care package in the person's home is possible but would prove too expensive for most people.

Care homes (or nursing homes, depending on the person's specific care needs) provide care in a homely environment with a mixture of care and nursing staff on-site 24 hours a day. A home (or chain of homes) could be run by the local authority, a charity, or a private enterprise. They vary widely in the quality of care provided and the standard of their facilities. In England, the Care Quality Commission regulates care and nursing homes. The Care Inspectorate regulates homes in Scotland. You can view the inspection reports online to help you decide which home is best for your relative. It also pays to visit homes you are interested in, meet the manager and staff, observe residents, and potentially speak to their family members. There are some excellent guides to things to consider and questions to ask published online by charities such as Age UK and Age Scotland.

Although not everyone with dementia will necessarily move to a care or nursing home, it tends to be a more positive experience when everyone – the person with dementia included – has been involved in considering the possibility and planning ahead. Outcomes are often less positive if arrangements are made under pressure. Unfortunately, many people with dementia move to care at short notice, often after admission to a hospital, where it becomes clear that returning home would be unsafe.

It can be difficult for everyone when a person with dementia moves into a care home. The person might find the transition to an unfamiliar environment distressing, particularly in the first few weeks or months. It also entails a significant change in lifestyle for families, especially when they have been responsible for much of the person's care and structured their time around them. It can take time to reconfigure routines and process conflicting emotions – like relief and guilt – the move into care might bring about. However, like accepting professional carers at home, the move can be a positive change. Family members might be able to enjoy spending time with the person as a spouse or child while care staff focus on the practical tasks. Some people with dementia – particularly those who lived alone previously – seem to temporarily improve after moving into care, perhaps because it is a relief for them. Many also benefit from regular company and stimulation.

Should someone with dementia avoid hospital admissions?

The benefits of a hospital admission must be weighed against possible harms. Harms of admission to hospital for someone with dementia include confusion, delirium, and possibly catching an infection. Unscheduled hospital admissions should be avoided unless absolutely necessary.

If a person with dementia does need to be admitted to a hospital, various things can help. First, do as much as possible to avoid them developing delirium, like ensuring that they have their glasses and hearing aids. Second, many hospitals have a facility where a dementia service can support the ward staff and the person with dementia. Alternatively, the ward team might have a dementia champion with specific knowledge about supporting people with dementia in hospital.

Finally, some hospitals use the 'Butterfly Scheme' to discreetly identify people with dementia who perhaps need extra time or help at mealtimes. These people use a different-coloured meal tray to alert ward staff.

What is the Newcastle model?

The 'Newcastle model' understands a person with dementia's stressed and distressed behaviours as communicating an 'unmet need'. The model emphasizes the importance of building a person-centred understanding of the person and their behaviour by getting to know them and their life experiences by speaking with the person, their family, and staff in the care home or hospital ward and completing structured assessments. By learning what is important to them, the ward team tries to understand why the person with dementia behaves in a particular way, producing a bio-psycho-social formulation. This formulation is discussed with the staff involved in the person's care and support, and strategies are agreed upon to meet the person's needs.

What about specialist dementia units?

A small number of people with advanced dementia have care needs that are too great for a care or nursing home. Instead, it can be necessary for them to be admitted to a specialist dementia unit in a hospital. Besides being based in a hospital, the main difference between these units and a care or nursing home is the increased provision of nursing staff. Someone might need a specialist dementia unit if they call out frequently and loudly, get distressed while receiving personal care – sometimes showing aggression or resistance requiring restraint – or show sexual disinhibition.

In most areas, admission to a specialist dementia unit is temporary. Reviewing the care plan and altering medications or psychological formulations (as in the Newcastle model) – in combination with the passage of time and the progression of the illness – can often lead to symptoms improving or resolving. However, some people remain in a specialist dementia unit until the end of their life.

Why might doors be locked? What about human rights?

Specialist dementia units – and some other wards – have locked doors to prevent someone with dementia from leaving unobserved and potentially coming to harm. Locking doors raises concerns about restrictions on a person's liberty and human rights.

The human rights of someone with dementia living somewhere behind a locked door is an area of much legal and academic debate. However, it is increasingly acknowledged that someone with dementia who lacks capacity to consent to be in a setting where they are not free to leave is being deprived of their liberty. A legal framework is needed to justify such a decision and protect their human rights.

Some people in such settings are detained under the relevant mental health act – for example the Mental Health (Care and Treatment) (Scotland) Act 2003, the Mental Health Act 2007 in England and Wales, or the Mental Health (Northern Ireland) Order 1986. Such legislation is also used when other additional powers are needed, such as a legal justification for restraint to provide essential personal care.

Alzheimer Scotland's 'Eight Pillars Model'

Alzheimer Scotland's 'Eight Pillars Model of Community Support' (Figure 15.1) builds on the 'Five Pillars Model' outlined earlier.

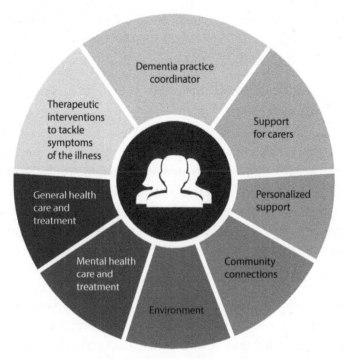

Figure 15.1 Alzheimer Scotland's Eight Pillar Model of Community Support

It addresses the needs of people with moderate-to-advanced dementia to enable them to live in their homes and communities for as long as possible and enjoy the best quality of life. The 'Advanced Dementia Practice Model' further extends the Eight Pillars, responding to people's needs in the most advanced phase of dementia.

The Eight Pillars are:

1 The dementia practice coordinator

Dementia affects every aspect of life, and each aspect of support must work in harmony to maximize the person's level of functioning. It is important to have someone responsible for ensuring that you can access all the support you need as and when required. In Scotland, this person is called the dementia practice coordinator – a named, skilled practitioner. This coordinator will liaise with everyone involved in your care, treatment, and support throughout your journey.

2 Therapeutic interventions to tackle the symptoms of dementia

A variety of therapeutic interventions can help the cognitive impairments, functional limitations, and behavioural problems caused by dementia: reality orientation, reminiscence therapy, cognitive stimulation therapy, and validation therapy aim to delay deterioration, enhance coping, maximize independence and improve quality of life. Medication to treat the symptoms of the illness is another intervention.

3 General health care and treatment

Regular medical reviews – usually by your GP – help ensure any health problems or illnesses are detected early and treated appropriately. Maintaining general wellbeing and physical health can improve your quality of life.

4 Mental health care and treatment

Regular mental health reviews help identify any problems, promote wellbeing, and treat illness. Psychiatrists, psychologists, nurses, and allied health professionals can assess, diagnose, and provide appropriate treatment. They can also support your family and carers to adapt to and cope with change, especially related to behavioural symptoms.

5 Personalized support

Personalized and flexible support is needed to help ensure you retain your independence, citizenship, and right to participate in society.

6 Support for carers

Your family and carers can benefit from education, skills training, coping strategies, and peer support. Their health and wellbeing should be considered independently of yours, including
their general and mental health, any need for a break from
caring, and the right to maintain and form their own social
connections.

7 Environment

Proactively identifying adaptations to your home environment
can support you to remain living in the community. Aids,
design changes, and assistive technology can help you remain
independent and make it easier to provide care and support at
home.

8 Community connections

Your quality of life, as well as that of your family and carers,
will be enhanced by continued contact with your existing social
networks and by establishing opportunities for peer support –
meeting others in a similar situation to you. Moreover, this
approach makes the most of the support you already have
around you – for example, other relatives, friends and neigh-
bours. It also helps you remain independent for longer.

16

How can I live well with dementia?

Am I still 'me' if I have a diagnosis of dementia?

The progress of dementia means that some things will inevitably change – the things you enjoy doing, how you express yourself, relate to others, and respond to and feel about your various experiences. However, with the right support and understanding, you can continue to express preferences and follow your interests, although this might be different from before. Your interests might change as you discover new preferences or begin to relate to people and places in new ways, as the 'me' you are now. But this 'me' is still continuous with who you have always been.

Should I tell other people about my diagnosis? Will people still accept me?

The general public is more aware of dementia than ever before, partly because of how common it is now. About 1 in 14 people aged 65 years and over have the illness in the UK – and 1 in 3 over 90 years. As a result, many families know someone living with dementia. As average life expectancy across the world continues to increase, so will the number of people affected by dementia.

Many communities have developed 'dementia-friendly' or 'dementia-inclusive' schemes. These aim to educate as many people as possible about what dementia is, the challenges it can present, and how to support people living with the disease in their everyday lives. Individuals can also become 'Dementia

Friends' (<www.dementiafriends.org.uk>) to learn more and show their support.

Consequently, the long-standing stigma attached to dementia is decreasing, and people living with the disease can generally remain active participants in their communities for longer. Shops and other public venues have often adapted their physical environments to ensure they are accessible. Employees are often more mindful of the challenges a person with dementia might experience and feel more confident to offer informed and sensitive support.

With this in mind, many people with dementia feel more able to be open about their diagnosis. Telling people about your diagnosis should not mean that your family or community excludes you. Nor should it mean that you are treated differently, in ways that limit your independence unnecessarily, or patronize you. By contrast, telling people about your diagnosis can help them to understand your experience and to speak with you about how they could support you.

What if my relatives do not accept my diagnosis?

Just as the person diagnosed can struggle to come to terms with the news, their relatives can find it difficult to accept that their loved one has dementia. Besides the many challenging symptoms, how you and your relatives relate to one another could change. You might become less curious, responsive, and empathetic. Whatever the length or nature of a relationship, some elements that define it will alter over time.

It can help to speak openly about your diagnosis and how you and the important people in your life feel about it. Seek out information to understand your condition and learn how all concerned can adapt to and cope with changes. Your local dementia charity can offer support and advice.

What if my family and friends don't know how to help?

Family and friends might find changes in their relationship with you hard to accept. They might worry that they will need to take on new responsibilities. Communication might be more challenging, and time together less immediately rewarding. Some people might be unsure what you can still do or what you and they should do together. For others, outdated notions that dementia is contagious persist. Such stigmas can lead people to stay away.

If your family and friends do stay away, your risk of becoming isolated increases. In turn, being isolated can affect your mental health and your carer's, result in a worse experience of dementia, and impact their ability to continue supporting you.

On the other hand, spending time with your family and friends can significantly improve your quality of life. Moreover, your carer might benefit from a break or doing things together with others.

If spending time with your family and friends is difficult, they can still be supportive by collecting food or prescriptions, preparing meals, or helping with forms and finances. These activities might take up your carer's time, sap their energy, and cause them to feel guilty for not being as focused on supporting you. Sometimes all family and friends need is an invitation to help and guidance on what they can do!

What can I do to plan ahead and have control over my future choices?

Dementia is a progressive illness, and most people will reach a stage where they can no longer make some decisions for themselves. However, no two dementia journeys are the same. For some people, things progress very slowly, but others experience a more rapid progression. There are a few ways in which you can plan for the future:

Powers of attorney

In most areas, you can nominate one or more people you trust to make decisions for you in the future if you cannot make such decisions for yourself. Powers of attorney can cover financial matters, property, and welfare decisions (including what care you should receive and where you should live). The lawyer setting up powers of attorney will help you specify the right powers for your situation. To nominate powers of attorney you must have legal decision-making capacity. If this is unclear, your lawyer may wish to speak to your doctor for their opinion.

In the first instance, the powers you have specified are registered but do not have any legal force until they are 'activated'. Usually, this is when you cannot make the decisions for yourself. Once activated, the person or people you have nominated now have the legal powers to make decisions as if you were making the decisions yourself. For this reason, decisions are scrutinized to ensure they are to your benefit.

Despite having the capacity to do so, you might be unsure about setting up a power of attorney. For some people with dementia, it feels like another step in an ongoing process of losing control.

For your carer

As a carer, it can help to introduce the idea gradually and to describe positive examples of how powers of attorney have benefited others. Many younger people, and people without dementia, have powers of attorney, too. Life is unpredictable, and it might be unexpectedly necessary. If you are to be an attorney but don't have the same legal document set up for yourself, it could help to suggest going through the process together. It might also help to explain that without powers of attorney, someone who does not know the person with dementia might be the one making decisions about them in the future.

If you decline to set up powers of attorney or lack the capacity to do so, you can apply for guardianship or conservatorship should you need legal powers in future. These powers achieve the same ends as powers of attorney but are more expensive and drawn-out processes that involve an eventual court order granting the legal powers.

Advance statement/living will

You can set out your thoughts and wishes for the future in an advance statement, advance directive, or living will. Depending on your location and preferences, this document can be more or less formal. In Scotland, for example, you can set out an advance statement to dictate how you would prefer to be treated should you become unwell and lack the capacity to decide at that time. The statement is witnessed and lodged in your medical records and with the relevant legal bodies. The doctors treating you must justify any treatment that conflicts with your advance statement. As such, it does not guarantee you will be treated as you set out but ensures that your views are taken into account.

Less formally, you can write an advance statement or living will, expressing your general views about your future care and treatment. However, it is important to consider that your current views of what you might want to happen in the future might not be how you feel when that future arrives. For example, you might imagine living with advanced dementia would be unthinkable. While dementia is an extremely challenging illness, many people living with dementia – even advanced dementia – can have an excellent quality of life.

Does being diagnosed with dementia mean that I have to stop...?

One reason that people with symptoms of dementia delay getting assessed is fear. Fear partly results from widespread mis-understandings about dementia. Simplistic media portrayals of people 'suffering from' dementia – suggesting a life of pain and victimhood – overlook the tremendous advances in understanding that have improved people's experience of living with the illness. In other words, it is possible to 'live well' with dementia, despite inevitable challenges. Slowly but surely, perceptions are changing, and many more nuanced television programmes and newspaper articles better reflect the multifaceted experiences of people with dementia.

The following three questions address some common fears about the repercussions of being diagnosed with dementia.

Will I be made redundant from my work?

While most people diagnosed with dementia are older than retirement age, an increasing number of people are diagnosed with 'young onset' or 'working age' dementia. In the UK, employers are legally obligated to explore reasonable and practicable adjustments to enable a person with dementia to continue to work. Depending on the nature of the specific role, adaptations to tasks, the work environment and working hours must be considered. Employers should also educate their broader workforce to increase awareness and understanding. Employers should take a sensitive and constructive approach that does not directly or indirectly discriminate against the person with dementia. If you are diagnosed with dementia and still working, speak to your employer about your work plans.

If you are diagnosed with dementia and are under 65 years old, you are likely to have a different set of responsibilities than someone diagnosed later in life. Beyond potentially working, you might have a mortgage or be looking after children or older relatives. Since dementia is largely perceived as a disease of older people, younger people with dementia often face more stigma and discrimination. Societal attitudes ('You can't have dementia if you can still function') and access to specialist services can be problematic. The latter might benefit younger people less because they are designed for those born in a previous era, who identify with different cultural touchstones, and who might be more physically frail.

Many organizations providing support to people with dementia have developed services to account for the unique circumstances people who are diagnosed at a younger age are likely to experience. Such services provide opportunities for the person with dementia and their family to meet people adapting to similar life changes.

Will I have to give up driving?

As with continuing to work, a diagnosis of dementia does not mean you must stop driving. However, the skills required to drive safely – such as focus and attention, reaction time, multi-tasking, memory, and decision-making – can be affected by dementia. As such, the point will come when you should stop. It is important to be aware of your driving ability and stop before becoming unsafe.

The thought of giving up driving can be an emotive issue. Driving is not only practical but about a sense of control and independence. People who cannot remember or accept their diagnosis might react badly to being told they must stop driving. They believe they are safe to continue. On the other hand, some people voluntarily surrender their licence because they know the potential risks to themselves and others.

It is a legal requirement that you or your family report the diagnosis to the relevant driving licensing authority as soon as possible. In the UK, not disclosing this information puts you at risk of incurring a substantial fine or being arrested. You must also report your diagnosis to your insurer or they could invalidate your insurance.

When reporting your diagnosis, you will need to share relevant medical information, which the licensing authority uses to determine whether you are safe to drive. The licensing authority will either: issue a temporary provisional licence; revoke your licence immediately; request further medical information; or stipulate a specialist on-road driving assessment before making a final decision.

If you are permitted to continue driving, you can keep yourself and others as safe as possible by: driving regularly and for only short periods on familiar routes during daylight hours; avoiding congestion; and minimizing distractions such as listening to the radio or music.

For your carer

As a carer, you can support a person who has to give up driving by listening to and acknowledging their concerns. Repeat the need to stop driving, but be clear that their illness is the reason and it is not a reflection of their previous abilities as a driver. Highlight alternative means of transport – buses, taxis, or specialist transport providers – as well as the potential benefits of stopping: reduced stress, saving money, and opportunities for more exercise and potentially meeting others. It might be necessary to remove the keys or sell or give their vehicle away, as seeing it parked outside might renew distress.

Some people with dementia will continue to drive without a valid licence, which can be dangerous as well as distressing for their family and friends. Under these circumstances, the family must contact the licensing authority, who will inform the local police about the situation. The person's doctor might break medical confidentiality and contact the licensing authority if their patient has refused to stop and is putting others at risk by continuing to drive.

Will I have to stop doing the things I enjoy?

Continuing to do things you enjoy is essential to living well with dementia. After diagnosis, you may not be able to act as if nothing has happened. However, the symptoms that led you to be assessed were already present when you last sang with your choir, visited the art gallery, or went shopping. You did not allow them to stop you from participating and enjoying those experiences. Life can continue while adapting to the present and thinking ahead to the future.

The dementia diagnosis is a clinical label for the symptoms you are experiencing. It helps explain what is happening, why, and what might happen over the months and years ahead. Getting a diagnosis is important because it can help you and others understand the condition and make adaptations over time to enable you to live well with and despite future challenges. A diagnosis also allows you to access appropriate services and support. The earlier you are diagnosed, the more insight and decision-making capacity you are likely to have, meaning you will have greater say over your future. Medication and treatments are more effective the earlier you start taking or receiving them.

At the same time, many people diagnosed with dementia at an early stage want to keep their distance from specialist services and anything labelled as being for 'people living with dementia'. You might take prescribed medication and check in with the nurse at intervals but remain connected to your usual occupations, interests, and hobbies. In time, as your symptoms impact your everyday life more, you might wish to also connect with specialist advice, information, and support. Alternatively, you might strike a balance between continuing to engage your current interests, seeking help, and meeting other people with dementia through groups and activities.

There is no right or wrong choice, but continuing to do what is normal and meaningful to you – despite your diagnosis – is essential to live well with dementia.

17

What changes should I make in my day-to-day life?

Would adopting a positive mental attitude help me?

A person with dementia once told Michael that the easiest thing to do after her diagnosis would have been to give up on herself. She could have stopped meeting up with friends, looking after her dog and house, going on holiday, and trying new things. However, she knew that to do so – to 'resign from life', as she put it – would mean a far worse experience of living with dementia.

To help her remain upbeat, she attributed the challenges she was experiencing to dementia – blaming dementia, not herself, if she made a mistake, for example. In so doing, she felt she was holding the disease at bay. She knew this effect would not last for ever. Still, she hoped that by adopting a positive mental attitude – and choosing to continue to live her life to the full – she would slow dementia's advance.

Some people with dementia will have neither the insight nor resilience to take this approach. Instead, family and friends can help create positive routines, including things to look forward to each day. By being positive, personalized, and aware of how they communicate, carers can help a person with dementia continue to enjoy meaningful experiences and maintain good mental health.

Are there benefits to following a routine?

Most people live by a set of routines – from when we wake up to when we return to bed. We often eat, work, exercise, and socialize at the same times and in the same places. We value routine because it lends life a degree of predictability and familiarity and helps us feel in control. We also like to break out of our routines now and then: to go out for a meal rather than cook; to walk a different route; to go on holiday. These daily patterns and rhythms are good for our mental wellbeing.

Following a routine can help limit the impact of short-term memory loss, decreased concentration span, and disorientation in space and time. Routine can also reduce anxiety about the changes you might be experiencing and help you feel more secure. It can also help your day pass with fewer moments of uncertainty and stress and improve communication and relationships with your family and friends.

A good routine will include a regular time for getting up and going to bed, as well as for meals and exercise, allow enough time for each activity, and incorporate your interests. It will also be flexible, factor in time to rest, and be mindful of when you are most alert and able. For example, you might find more stressful experiences (like shopping) easier earlier in the day, when you are less tired.

Does what I eat and drink affect my experience of dementia?

As dementia progresses, many people find it harder to eat well and stay hydrated. The consequences of poor diet and dehydration are many: you could experience weight gain or loss, the onset or deterioration of other health conditions (diabetes, cardiovascular disease, etc.), constipation, urinary tract infections, low mood, and low energy.

The most common challenges associated with eating and drinking that result from dementia, and some possible responses, are:

- **Changing tastes and appetite.** Your taste buds can be affected by dementia. You might prefer different flavours and need to adjust your diet to continue eating nutritious foods.
- **Memory loss.** You might forget to eat or overeat because you don't remember already having done so. If you live alone and don't have support with meals, you could use a smartphone or digital assistant (such as an Amazon Alexa) to remind you to eat. You could record when and what you have eaten each day. It can help to have water bottles visible where you spend most of your time at home.
- **Communication difficulties.** You might find it more difficult to express when you are hungry or thirsty. Following a routine can help you eat at regular mealtimes. Should you live with your carer or have other support, they can periodically check if you want anything to eat or drink. They might also observe patterns in your behaviour that indicate you are hungry.
- **Visual perception.** You might not always recognize food as food. Red dinner plates and utensils have been shown to not only optimize colour contrast with most food – helping with recognition – but grab the attention and stimulate appetite. When eating with other people, they could describe what's on your plate (and your cutlery, glass, etc.) to reduce the chances of you mistaking one thing for another.
- **Motor control.** Handling cutlery, cutting up and moving food to the mouth can all become more complicated. To help, you could purchase adapted cutlery or eat more finger foods, or other people could demonstrate how or support you to eat.
- **Poor concentration.** You might feel restless and find it hard to sit long enough to finish a meal. It can help to take a walk before a meal and to minimize distractions – such as the

television or radio – while eating. Eating with others where possible could also help you remain focused. Easy-to-eat foods require less concentration.

- **Difficulty chewing and swallowing**. Chewing and your automatic swallow function might be less consistent as dementia impacts the parts of the brain responsible. In such a situation, you will need support from other people. They can prompt you to chew and swallow. Consideration should be given to the type of food provided, and you should only have small amounts of food in your mouth at a time. You should seek advice and support from a speech and language therapist.
- **Poor mouth care**. Looking after your oral health can help you avoid mouth or gum infections, maintain the ability to eat, and improves taste. Brush your teeth (or clean your dentures) twice daily, and have regular dental check-ups.

How important is it to sleep well?

People with dementia often talk of having 'good days and bad days' and not always being able to predict in advance which will occur. A key factor can be the amount and quality of sleep the night before. Your sleep can be affected by:

- changes to your body clock
- levels of the sleep hormone melatonin reduce as you age
- needing to go to the toilet more often overnight
- side effects of medication
- signs of restlessness such as repetitive leg movements
- eating or drinking stimulants such as sugar and caffeine close to bedtime
- sleeping during the day to compensate for sleep lost overnight.

Tiredness can exacerbate the ordinary symptoms of dementia: recalling short-term memories, thought processes, word finding, and the sequencing and motor control skills required to carry out practical tasks. Your mood will likely be lower and more prone to fluctuations.

The following tips might help you sleep better:

- Spend time outside in natural daylight, walking or in the garden. Even sitting by a window exposed to natural daylight can help improve sleep quality.
- If daytime naps are needed, try to do so earlier, and limit them to no more than an hour so that it is less likely to affect your sleep at night.
- Eat more at lunch and less at night. It is also helpful to reduce your consumption of caffeine, sugar, and other stimulants, including alcohol.
- If you drink close to bedtime, camomile tea or a warm, milk-based drink can be calming.
- 18–21 degrees Celsius (64–70 degrees Fahrenheit) is a comfortable room temperature for most people. To adapt, change your nightwear and bedding depending on temperature/season. If you feel cold, you could use a hot water bottle or electric blanket to warm the bed.
- Check you have a comfortable pillow and mattress.
- If you wear continence products, ensure they are dry before bed.
- Motion-sensitive night lights can help you orient and find your way to the bathroom.
- A dementia clock can help you orient yourself if you wake up confused.
- Black out the room as much as possible to make it easier to get back to sleep.

Is it a good idea to exercise?

A positive routine will incorporate exercise; however, you should consider your physical capacity and adjust your activity accordingly. A total of half an hour's gentle exercise (which can be taken in short bursts) most days is a good target.

Many people with dementia will continue the exercises they enjoyed before diagnosis. Others take up new forms of exercise, and there are many opportunities aimed at 'older' people that are dementia inclusive, such as walking football. As well as being more active you will meet people through taking part.

Short, regular periods of exercise with a carer or friend can benefit your physical and mental health. Even a short walk in the morning and afternoon can help structure your day and provide a change of scene.

If you experience difficulties with strength, balance, and coordination, gentle seated exercises can be an effective alternative.

Is it still worth doing activities?

People with dementia can still engage in meaningful and enjoyable activities. The fact that you might not always remember the whole experience does not mean it was pointless. Because of the changes of dementia, if someone asked you about an activity you have participated in – even immediately afterwards – you might only be able to offer a general response. How the activity made you *feel* tends to stay with you for longer. Emotional memories are more protected from dementia than memories of facts. There is great value in continuing to engage in socially and mentally stimulating activities.

Spending time with others and participating in activities – such as singing, craft, dance, baking, storytelling, and art – produces immediate short-term benefits. You might feel more engaged and communicative while participating and after the experience.

In addition, positive emotional memories can improve your mood and make it more likely you will repeat the experience. This virtuous cycle of participation, stimulation, and enjoyment can help you remain positive and engaged, reducing the likelihood of apathy or depression. By contrast, if you withdraw and become isolated, you might enter a vicious cycle of stress and distress, exacerbating the ordinary symptoms of dementia.

Not all people with dementia will be interested in or enjoy social activities. Keeping up in conversation, word finding, and hearing difficulties can put people off spending time with others. Being more sensitive to noise and other stimulation can result in sensory overload, causing anxiety and agitation.

For your carer

As a carer, be mindful that the person with dementia will not always initiate activities. They might not know about opportunities in the community or engage in pastimes at home. Sharing information about what is available or leaving crosswords, jigsaws, or knitting out might not always be enough. The person with dementia could require encouragement, reminders, transport, and companionship to start and then continue to attend a group. At home, it might be necessary to spend time demonstrating an activity or even doing it together to bring it to life. Choosing activities that are not too challenging but give a feeling of accomplishment and satisfaction can also help.

Can reminiscing help?

A helpful way of thinking about memory loss is the 'bookcase analogy'. Imagine that your memory is a bookcase: each shelf represents a decade's worth of memories, each memory stored in a unique book. The top shelves are your most recent memories. The shelves in between are your middle years – when you started your first job, met your spouse or partner, might have had children, and so on. The shelves towards the foot of the bookcase are your teenage and childhood years.

In this analogy, dementia is a strong wind blowing against and rocking the bookcase from side to side, causing the books nearest the top – your most recent memories – to fall and be borne away. Being lower, the books nearer the middle and foot of the bookcase resist the wind longer, and the memories stored here can still be recalled. Indeed, they might take on new clarity in the relative absence of shorter-term memories.

For this reason, you might be able to talk in great detail about the events of your formative years but not always remember what you had for breakfast. People without dementia also store long-term memories but they are obscured by short-term necessities such as remembering appointments and to pay bills.

Memory loss is not uniform; memories can come and go, often triggered by different conversations, sounds, smells, or objects. A memory not there one moment might return minutes, hours, or days later.

Reminiscence can be particularly effective if you are mixing up your past and present, perhaps believing you are at an earlier stage of their life. You might refer to former work routines or tasks as if you are currently engaged in them.

For your carer

As carer, listen for references to particular episodes from the person's past, which can be clues as to where they might be on their 'timeline'. Rather than challenging and potentially upsetting them, it can be beneficial to enter that reality with the person, talking about their memories. What did they do? What did they enjoy? Who did they work with? Reminiscing in this way can affirm their identity, which might feel increasingly fragmented as dementia progresses.

Using photographs, objects, or visiting places that were (and remain) important to them can maintain a connection between their past and present and help differentiate between the two.

Working together on recording the person with dementia's life story can be a positive, meaningful project that values their experiences. It also allows people who do not know the person well – such as paid carers and other professionals – to start good, personalized conversations. When someone is admitted to a hospital or moves into a care home, sharing their life story with staff can help make the transition easier.

Engaging with the past might sometimes cause the person distress. Not all memories are positive, and reminiscence risks reliving difficult experiences. Exploring positive memories can be difficult if the person contrasts them with present challenges.

How does being in pain affect dementia?

Dementia itself does not cause pain, but people with dementia might experience more pain in general because they are generally older, may have other health conditions, and are at an increased risk of falling, accidents, and injury.

People with dementia are not less sensitive to pain. However, because of changes in cognition and communication skills, people might be less able to say they are in pain. This can complicate accurate diagnosis and treatment. Carers should observe non-verbal signs of pain such as changes in gait, restricted movements, holding or rubbing body parts, and changes in mood and behaviour. Health professionals also have to use a broader range of diagnostic tools to identify pain than they might in someone without dementia.

Even if a person with dementia can communicate effectively, other factors can lead to pain being underreported. These can include depression, fear of requiring surgery, hospitalization, or being moved into long-term care, misperceptions about the effects of medication, and cultural, religious, and gender differences.

Untreated pain results in unnecessary suffering, can contribute to depression, and exacerbate the ordinary symptoms of dementia. Uncharacteristic behaviours, such as agitation and aggression, can be caused by pain but are often attributed to something else. As a result, people can be prescribed inappropriate medications, including antipsychotics, with potentially serious side effects.

Untreated pain can cause people to withdraw further from meaningful activities and social interaction. It may also impair mobility, increasing the risk of falls and other injuries.

How can I manage my general health?

People with dementia must have access to diagnosis, treatment, and care services for other illnesses. About three in four people with dementia have at least one other health condition. These could include high blood pressure (hypertension), diabetes, stroke or transient ischemic attack (TIA), coronary heart disease (CHD), depression, chronic obstructive pulmonary disease (COPD), or asthma. Diagnosing other health conditions in people with dementia can be complicated, particularly as dementia becomes more advanced.

Scheduling a regular appointment with your GP and attending specialist clinics as required is important. Unmanaged, these conditions could cause problems in their own right and also exacerbate the ordinary symptoms of dementia.

A routine that includes eating well, staying hydrated, regular exercise, and good sleep can help reduce the likelihood of infections, fractures, and pressure sores. Appropriate medication can help manage persistent pain and optimize general health. Having a system – or accepting help or supervision, if necessary – to ensure you take medication as prescribed can also be helpful.

18

How can I best support a person with dementia?

We generally refer to 'people living with dementia' and 'carers' to separate people with a diagnosis from those who, over time, assume more responsibility for helping the former maintain a good quality of life. Some services and support, as well as some financial benefits, are aimed at one rather than the other. However, such labels can overlook that carers – often spouses, children, siblings – are also 'living with dementia'. They, too, experience the practical and emotional challenges of dementia. It is also true that many people diagnosed with dementia can be carers for another person.

Many carers tell us that caring is not what they had planned for retirement. The sentiment is repeated by those raising young children, trying to hold down a job, and/or managing their own physical or mental health difficulties. Just as each person with dementia has a history, interests, and desires, so does each carer. Any carer, regardless of how they feel about the person they are caring for or how well suited they are to caring, will find aspects of the experience stressful and upsetting. At the same time, many carers, although they would change the course of events if they could, find the experience of caring rewarding and satisfying. They know they are supporting someone through potentially the most challenging and ultimately terminal stage of their life.

How can I see the person, not the dementia?

The person diagnosed with dementia is the same person you have always known. No matter how much dementia impacts their present and future, or alters their recollection of the past, they remain a wife, husband, mother, father, brother, sister, or friend. The person will still have interests and passions, fears and anxieties, hopes and ambitions. Understanding their experience and feelings is key to supporting them to live well with dementia.

There are numerous suggestions for supporting a person with dementia – this book included – but no universal formula. The approaches which work will be informed by what you know about who they are. Supporting someone is a process of trial and error that starts with communication – speaking with the person, learning how they feel, what they want, and what would help them. If dementia has impacted verbal communication, observe their body language, facial expressions, and behaviour. Doing so will show you whether your actions are supportive or causing distress. Much of what are sometimes labelled – wrongly – 'challenging' behaviours result from unmet needs: a person being hungry or tired, too hot or cold, or under-stimulated.

Use what you know about the person to motivate them. If they did not enjoy group activities before dementia, they might still feel that way now. However, if they were interested in football, fashion, or film, they might want to join in a themed activity.

Remember that the person with dementia you care for is still the person you have been married to or brought up by, with their unique life story, interests, and desires. However much change the disease brings about, the person does not become their dementia any more than a person with a tumour becomes their cancer.

Try to empathize with how they might be feeling. Speak with, listen to, and observe them. Learn more about dementia by reading and speaking to other carers and professionals. Use this knowledge to inform how you care.

How can I make sense of how the person I care for feels and behaves?

When you are tired, stressed, and worried, it will not always be easy. Try to keep in mind that the behaviours that you find challenging are a result of the disease, not the person. That's not to say that everything was perfect pre-diagnosis – some frustrating character traits are definitely not exclusive to dementia! However, a person's inability to remember and concentrate, among other things, is not deliberate. They are not trying to wind you up and are not likely to be manipulative or deceitful, or have 'selective memory'. People with dementia are usually unable to think through the complexities required to manipulate others. Instead, the person might be filling in gaps in their memory or altering parts of the story because they can't recall what happened.

A person with dementia's behaviour may appear challenging but it is important to remember that they are trying to communicate their feelings and needs. As such, behaviours are usually triggered by something: pain, boredom, frustration; being too hot or hungry, or needing to use the toilet; or their perception of how the people around them are treating them and communicating.

Behaviours that carers can find 'challenging' include:

- the person constantly moving around (possibly looking for the toilet, their room, out of boredom, or needing to exercise)
- repetitive questioning (because they can't remember having asked before or the answer you gave, or otherwise betraying anxiety)
- searching and hoarding (because they can't remember where they left something or else to hold on to, protect, and practise control over something – money, for example – when feeling a general loss of control)
- wanting to tidy up or set the table (because it is a skill they can still put to use).

Try not to take behaviours personally or take out your frustration on the person with dementia. Instead, try to identify their unmet needs and any patterns (such as the time of day they become distressed), and any early indicators that their mood is changing. Being proactive can potentially nip things in the bud and help you both remain emotionally well.

When a person with dementia behaves in a way that you find challenging, it can help to ask yourself if the behaviour is actually a problem. If so, who is it a problem for and why? Some behaviours are coping mechanisms for the person with dementia but affect carers because what they are doing does not reflect how they were before dementia.

What is the ABC model?

If a particular behaviour is a problem for the person with dementia or those caring for them, the ABC, or 'Antecedent–Behavior–Consequence', model, provides a framework to help identify the cause(s) of the behaviour. You can then offer appropriate support to help the person with dementia return to a calm state. You can also develop strategies to reduce the likelihood of the same or similar behaviours happening again or the amount of distress experienced if it does.

Using the ABC model is especially helpful if there are multiple carers – unpaid or paid – as it can improve the consistency of care provided. Changes in a person's behaviour might indicate a progression in their dementia or highlight underlying conditions (including pain, constipation, or infections) which can exacerbate the ordinary symptoms of dementia.

The ABC model works as follows:

A = Antecedent

What happened leading up to the person with dementia becoming distressed? You might identify the cause or trigger for their distress by identifying the antecedent. What is it that led the person to act in this way? Common antecedents include:

- situations in which the person is fearful, embarrassed, or frustrated
- where they perceive that they are being mistreated or misunderstood by others
- environmental factors such as noise or commotion
- unmet needs such as pain, discomfort, needing to go to the toilet, hunger, and boredom – difficulty communicating needs can mean that distressed behaviour might be the only way to express how they are feeling.

B = Behaviour

What happened? Take note of specific and relevant details. Typical behaviours include shouting, swearing, and striking out. You should also note when the behaviour occurred, how long it lasted, and any indication that it was about to happen. Signs could include restlessness, reduced eye contact, a verbal instruction to stop, or less communication than usual. Record what you did to stop or reduce the person's experience of distress, as well as any approaches that had the opposite effect.

C = Consequence

What were the consequences of how they behaved? How did the person feel afterwards? Did they calm down immediately or remain upset? Was anybody physically hurt or injured?

Should I let the person I care for know when they've made a mistake?

We are all likely to feel embarrassed if someone points out our mistakes. Owing to changes in memory, sequencing, decision-making, and communication skills, a person with dementia will – compared to what we consider normal – make 'mistakes': putting keys in the fridge, leaving the front door open, or forgetting to pay in the shop.

Pointing out their mistakes will not alter future behaviour, or even reduce the chances of the same mistakes happening again. Instead, correction can highlight the challenges the person is experiencing and make their mistakes and behaviours more of an issue than they need to be. Doing so can imply that the person forgets on purpose and that they will stop making the same mistake if you remind them enough.

While it can be hard to accept mistakes from a person we know to have been very capable, bear in mind that they might not even remember having made a mistake, so will likely deny responsibility.

Similarly, a story that the person with dementia tells might not be entirely factual. While their current experience and perception could be very different from yours, it will feel, to them, equally valid. Instead of correcting their story – which could hurt their feelings, lead to an argument, and even make them communicate less (for fear of being wrong) – it might be emotionally better for you both to broadly go along with what they are saying.

It will not always be possible to remain calm, respond positively, or decide to accept what the person with dementia says, whether true or not. Each of us is different, and few possess infinite reserves of patience and resilience: you are human, not an automaton! Nor is your relationship a blank slate, wiped clean at the point of diagnosis. You have a history together that, for better or worse, will also shape how you respond to stressful situations in the present. There will be times when you lose your temper, raise your voice, and let out your frustrations on the person you are caring for, only to feel guilty for doing so. It is normal for carers to respond in ways that don't always improve things. Forgiving yourself when this happens is important.

It can help to speak about how you feel to other family members, friends, and local voluntary carer organizations.

In short, then, we suggest 'picking your battles'. Take a moment to reflect on whether the behaviour is a problem, and if so, who for and why. It will sometimes be necessary not to go along with what the person is doing or saying – for example, if the person is a risk to themselves or others, or if what they say could potentially hurt you or other people emotionally. Otherwise, to prevent causing the person with dementia needless emotional distress, which will take a toll on you, avoid pointing out mistakes or correcting behaviours and stories.

What is the best way to communicate with the person I care for?

Effective communication between a carer and a person with dementia is essential to sustaining a positive relationship that enables rather than disables the person with the condition.

How well a person with dementia can communicate will depend on changes in memory, language processing, word finding, and rational thinking. People with dementia can lose their train of thought and not be able to finish a sentence. They can call objects and people by the wrong word. They can take longer to understand what others are saying to them and respond.

Should carers be aware of the challenges the person with dementia is experiencing, they can help the person feel heard, understood, and valued. Doing so can reduce their frustration at not always being able to say what they want. As with many symptoms of dementia, it can help to think about how we feel when we occasionally say the wrong thing or struggle to find the words we want to use. How exasperating it must be when there is repeatedly a difference between what you want and what you are able to say! Not being understood is one cause of aggressive verbal and non-verbal behaviours people with dementia sometimes direct at carers.

Here are some things to consider when communicating with a person with dementia. How relevant each suggestion is will depend on your relationship with the person and how well they communicate. Always communicate with them as an individual. Try to avoid patronizing them. Talking loudly will not make you easier to understand. Doing so will likely make the person with dementia feel uncomfortable and embarrassed.

What should I think about before communicating with a person with dementia?

Before communicating, think about the environment: are you somewhere quiet and well-lit with few distractions (such as the television on in the background)? If you want to talk about something important, have you thought about what you plan to say, and do you have enough time not to feel rushed?

Put yourself in the person with dementia's position: from what you know about the person's typical mood and behaviour, is it a good time of day to talk? Are their other needs met, or might they be hungry, in pain, or need to use the toilet?

Position yourself so that you are at the same level as them and can make eye contact. Is your face lit so the person can see your facial expressions? Are you close enough to hear while respecting the person's need for personal space?

Professor Alison Wray from Cardiff University has produced a helpful series of videos on communication and dementia, which can be found at: <www.youtube.com/channel/UC6kMlO8mkB09GNCLm1zbaHQ>

How should I speak to a person with dementia?

Speaking clearly, calmly, and potentially more slowly than usual allows the person time to process what you are saying and respond. Short, simple sentences with only one key point can also help the person process and follow the conversation. Remember, too, that you are having a conversation. Instead of interviewing the person – asking question after question – offer your thoughts, opinions, and feelings, and reflect on what they are saying.

By keeping your body language open and relaxed, the person with dementia is more likely to feel the same. Similarly, laugh together about any misunderstandings. Well-timed, sensitive moments of light-heartedness can help defuse stressful situations.

What should I say, and what should I not?

Try to avoid asking too many questions or questions that are complicated. It can also help to avoid asking direct questions that challenge the person to remember information, particularly about the recent past. The person might be more able to talk confidently about how they feel/felt or share a view or opinion. If what the person says is not the same as what you understand to be true or false, try to avoid directly contradicting them. Never ridicule what they have said or patronize them. Avoid mentioning 'mistakes' the person has made or pointing out unusual behaviours. The chances are the person will have forgotten and, as such, might feel embarrassed and even defensive, which can lead to renewed distress and bad feeling between you.

Sticking to one topic at a time can help a person remain focused and engaged. Similarly, keeping conversations short and regular will be less tiring and mean the person is less likely to lose concentration.

If the person does not understand what you are saying, rephrase and simplify rather than repeating exactly. You could consider using non-verbal communication such as gestures or visual cues (e.g. objects and pictures) to help if appropriate.

What is active listening and how can it help?

Active listening is listening to and observing the verbal and non-verbal communication of the person you are interacting with. It means engaging with what they say and how they feel. Using facial expressions and body language that match the emotions of the person with dementia can help the person feel listened to and understood. You should check you have understood the person speaking by rephrasing what you have heard back to them.

Observing the facial expressions and body language of the person you are speaking to, you can check they understand what you are saying and see how they feel. You can then adapt how you communicate.

While the person should have time to process what you are saying and respond, it is OK to speak again if a long pause makes them uncomfortable or embarrassed.

There might not always be a solution to a worry or concern that the person shares with you. However, always respect their right to express their feelings. Simply listening and showing that you care can be very reassuring.

Try not to presume that you know what the person intends to say by finishing their sentences. Allow the person to speak for themselves as much as possible; offer encouragement where necessary but do not second-guess their wishes, feelings, and opinions.

What about body language and physical contact?

As dementia progresses, non-verbal cues become a more integral part of communication. Closed body language, such as folded arms or worried facial expression, might suggest that you don't want to be with the person or are unsure how to interact. By contrast, an open stance and relaxed expression can help the person feel at ease and involved in the conversation. At the same time, try to ensure your facial expressions match what you are saying. For example, should it be necessary to share upsetting news, it might be insensitive to appear upbeat and unempathetic.

Used appropriately, physical touch can offer comfort and reassurance – holding the person's hand or laying your hand on their arm while talking. However, each person will respond to touch differently, so be aware of their body language and what they say to ensure they are comfortable.

Should I do everything for the person I care for?

With the best intentions, many carers assume more control over and responsibility for the person with dementia's life and affairs. They might *do for* rather than *do with* because it is hard to watch someone they care for struggle, or it is easier or more efficient without their help. Over time this will, in most cases, become necessary. However, especially in the earlier stages of dementia, removing a sense of purpose can cause the person to lose skills and confidence sooner than they would otherwise. It can also negatively impact their mood and motivation.

For example, a person with dementia might be unable to make a whole meal from scratch. However, not involving the person at all could make them feel useless. They might begin to believe they are incapable and withdraw, refuse to help with jobs at home and take part in social opportunities. Such a chain of events can accelerate the person's dementia.

The overriding experience of dementia can quickly become one of loss. This is not inevitable. A person with dementia who is supported to remain active and independent is likely to have greater self-belief and be motivated to use their strengths and skills for longer.

It is important to avoid talking about the person with dementia as if they are not there, telling others about the challenges you are going through. Whatever their level of verbal understanding, the person will pick up on some meaning directly from the words you use and some from how you say them. Instead, include them in the conversation. They might not always have a full grasp of the details but are likely to have an opinion and know how they feel about the topic.

You might need to put more thought into where to go, what to do, and even who to do it with, but supporting the person with dementia to maintain their relationships and participate in social activities, hobbies, and interests will help them feel 'normal' and valued. For many people with dementia, remembering what happened is more difficult than remembering how they felt. Some carers wonder if supporting the person they care for to be involved in things is worthwhile because they can't recall what was talked about or who they were with. However, the emotional memories that reflect how the person felt about what they did remain strong. Positive emotional memories can mean they are in a better mood and communicate more with their carers afterwards.

Should we spend time apart?

People with dementia can also feel constrained by their carers. There is an understandable focus on the need for carers to have time to themselves to recharge or follow their interests. However, people with dementia also benefit from the opportunity to be independent and express themselves freely.

At the Dementia Cafés that Michael and his Alzheimer Scotland colleagues run, half an hour is spent together as a group of people living with dementia and their family and carers. For the following hour, the group splits into a therapeutic activity group for those with dementia and a peer support group for carers in separate rooms.

The idea is that carers require a space to talk openly and honestly about their practical and emotional experience supporting their relatives. Hopefully, they will feel understood by each other as people living through a similar situation.

In the other room, people with dementia participate in an activities group. Michael notices that many participants are more confident and communicative when given time and a safe, supportive space to share their experiences with others in a similar situation. It can be a relief to speak without worrying whether they have told a story correctly or are being judged by others.

In short, finding opportunities for experiences apart can be advantageous to both the carer and the person with dementia.

Is it a good idea to help the person I care for make choices and feel in control?

It is normal to want to feel in control of our lives. To be able to make choices and decisions that affect our day-to-day experience independently, or, at the very least, to be considered an equal partner in a relationship. As their symptoms progress, people with dementia can lose this sense of being in control. As such, the onus can be on carers to support the person to make as many choices for themselves as they can.

Choices range from everyday decisions about when to get up, what to eat and wear, and how to spend time, to life-changing deliberations about relationships, finances, health, and welfare. Gradually, a person's capacity to make choices in their 'best interests' will become more complicated. They might be medically assessed as no longer having the capacity to make certain choices – perhaps about where they are safe to live, whether a hospital admission is necessary, or a medical procedure permitted. Before this point is reached, it can be helpful to put a legal mechanism such as powers of attorney in place to allow other trusted people to become involved.

However, to be clear, being assessed as lacking capacity does not mean that the person is incapable of making any choices. Wherever possible, they should be asked their views on the significant decisions that affect them and be supported to make everyday choices. Some people might find open-ended choices too much. As such, you can help day-to-day decision-making by offering a limited number of options based on what you know about the person's preferences.

What changes could I make to the person's home?

Most people with dementia prefer to stay in their own homes and live as independently as possible for as long as possible. A growing field of dementia-friendly design developed in line with the lived experience of people with dementia is helping make this a reality. Practical, often low-cost adaptations to the home environment can significantly prolong the length of time people can live where they feel most happy and secure.

People with dementia must be involved in conversations about their home environment, and ideally, at an early stage of the illness, to help them make informed choices about their present and future needs and plans. Conversations should focus on what the person can do and what, with the correct adaptations, they could continue to do.

Any changes should respect the person's preferences and tastes as much as possible. It can do more harm than good if the home environment is no longer familiar – if, for example, the person's home is made to resemble a clinical setting in the name of safety.

Safety

Safety will always be a key concern, especially if the person with dementia lives alone. Occupational therapy and fire service assessments look in detail at the home environment from this standpoint. They might install, for example, grab rails, alarms, and sensors. Other safety measures to take include:

- checking the thermostat regularly, particularly as the seasons change, to prevent the person feeling too hot or cold
- reducing the hot water temperature settings to prevent scalding
- keeping important telephone numbers by the house phone and/or stored in the person's mobile in case of emergency
- installing socket covers and control valves so that the person doesn't accidentally turn on or off appliances, heating, gas, and so on
- ensuring the person can use door handles and lock the property without any issues.

An environment that is safe and accessible for a person with dementia will be safe and accessible for everyone. However, many households are home to more than the person with dementia. They might be multi-generational and need to accommodate various needs and preferences.

Decluttering

'Decluttering' the home environment can be a quick win. Carers can help create a more relaxed, less visually distracting, or overwhelming space and make the things the person uses most often easier to find. It is sensible to remove or replace obvious trip hazards, such as rugs and pieces of furniture. However, objects of sentimental value can 'store' memories and trigger positive associations. To remove them might take away one means of connecting with a particular memory.

Lighting

Good lighting can help people with dementia see well and feel oriented in space. Natural light also helps with orientation in time. Lighting reduces shaded areas and shadows which can help avoid misperceptions and illusions. Installing dimmer switches gives the person control over the level of light they need. Touch-lit lamps can be less fiddly than those operated via a switch. At night, a dark bedroom can improve sleep length and quality, and sensor lights that come on when the person moves around are helpful if they need to get up to go to the bathroom.

Furniture and furnishings

By contrasting the colour of furniture with the walls and floor, the person with dementia will be better able to identify light switches, their bed, table, chairs, and lamps, making them easier to use. Typically, chairs with arms that are not too low are easier to get into and out of. Stripes and strong patterns can cause confusion and disorientation and are best used sparingly. Likewise, as symptoms intensify, paintings, artworks, and mirrors can also be confusing. They can be covered or removed if necessary. Retaining the basic layout of each room can help the person remember and navigate their surroundings more easily.

Flooring

Some people with dementia begin to shuffle, not fully lifting their feet from the floor. Strength and balance can also decrease. Both changes mean that trips and falls are more likely. At home, uneven floors or mats increase the risk still further. Issues with visual perception might make shiny floors appear wet or slippery, and dark-coloured surfaces look like holes. Plain, non-shiny floors will be more straightforward to move across. Contrasting the colour of the stairs with the surrounding walls, and laying a bright strip of tape on the lip of the step, can make going up and down safer.

Using the bathroom

Affixing a sign showing a picture of a toilet and the word 'Toilet' to the door at eye level, or leaving the door open, can make it easier to find the bathroom. Leave the bathroom light on at night or use sensor lights that respond to movement. To prevent the person with dementia from becoming trapped, adjust any locking mechanism to ensure it is always possible to open the bathroom door from the outside. Contrasting the colour of the toilet seat and lid from the rest of the toilet (or even removing the lid) can help the person feel less anxious about finding the toilet and reduce the potential for accidents. To help them use the bath, shower, and toilet, you could install grab rails that contrast with the colour of the wall. Fitting taps with traditional mechanisms marked hot and cold, and a handle flush toilet can help the person know how to operate both. Flood prevention plugs release water from the bath or sink if they forget to turn the tap off, and some plugs change colour to indicate if the water is too hot. Keeping only essential products in the bathroom reduces clutter and the potential for disorientation and confusion. Using non-slip mats minimizes the risk of falls.

Navigating the home environment

Affixing a picture/label to the outside of cupboards, drawers, doorways, the fridge, and so on, to indicate the contents, can help the person with dementia find what they are looking for. Likewise, a picture/label affixed to the door into a room can help them orient themself and reduce anxieties about getting lost or confused. Alternatively, transparent doors allow the person to see what is stored inside. Removing cupboard doors where they cover washing machines, dishwashers, and fridge freezers can also help. Decluttering surfaces and reducing stored contents can make the most frequently used items easier to identify. You can help the person with dementia locate the things they regularly use (such as keys, phone, glasses, and wallet/purse) by encouraging the habit of keeping them in one place.

Dementia can mean that some people are hypersensitive to noise. Positioning noisy appliances – such as a washing machine – at a distance from where they are likely to spend most of their time can reduce the impact on thinking and language-processing, as can turning off the television or radio when they are not the person's focus. Similarly, carpets and curtains or fabric blinds are better at absorbing sound than laminate floors and wooden blinds.

Not all adaptations will be practical. For example, a three-storey house with external steps might not be safely habitable throughout the illness. Sometimes it is necessary and beneficial to discuss housing options sooner rather than later, giving the person with dementia the best opportunity to adjust to a new environment.

Could technology help make life easier?

Technology is an inescapable fact of contemporary life; we use it all the time. A diagnosis of dementia does not mean that a person must stop benefiting from the range of available aids. Using 'assistive technology' can enable a person to remain independent for longer. It can help people stay connected to family and friends, stay well physically, and feel secure at home and safe in their community.

It is sometimes assumed that people with dementia cannot learn new things. However, with repetition and appropriate memory strategies, it is possible to develop and retain new skills for some time, even as cognition declines in other ways.

Moreover, we already see the current generation of people diagnosed with dementia in their sixties and seventies confidently using mobile phones and the internet to communicate, find information, and follow their interests. In the early stages of living with dementia, it is normal for these skills to remain and can help people handle everyday challenges. This trend will only increase over time as future generations age and develop dementia.

A wide range of electronic and non-electronic technology is available to people with dementia, some designed to solve common problems and some existing technology repurposed to aid people with dementia. It is beyond the scope of this book to detail all the technology that can help – and, given the speed with which new technology develops, we would soon seem outdated! – but can recommend the following website produced by the Digital Team at Alzheimer Scotland:

The most important thing to consider is whether any given piece of technology is the right one for this person. Speaking to other people with dementia and their carers, reading or watching reviews, consulting dementia technology specialists (such as dementia charities and occupational therapists), and trying out different technologies can help find the most suitable aids.

The person with dementia should be the one to make decisions about the technology they use. If they lack the capacity to consent, the person should still be as involved as possible in making an informed choice. When thinking about future plans, it can be helpful for the person with dementia to consider the role they would like technology to take in their ongoing care and support as their needs change.

It is also worth noting that some assistive technology can be expensive. It can be a good idea to explore renting or acquiring technology second-hand.

Is it still possible to enjoy time with the person I care for?

It may sound cliché, but it is important to take things one day at a time when living with dementia and caring for someone with the illness. Try to continue participating in and enjoying the things that are meaningful to you both for as long as possible.

As a carer, understanding more about the type of dementia the person you care for has been diagnosed with gives you an idea of how the disease might progress and can help identify concerns. It can also help to plan for the future while the person can still make their own decisions. However, it is equally vital to be in the moment and focus on what is positive and possible rather than worrying too much about what might be ahead. Some carers record the good things that happen each day. There will be many, but they are easily forgotten about when stressed and exhausted. When things are particularly hard-going, looking back at this record can remind you that it's not all bad and help you keep going.

19

Self-care as a carer

How can I look after a person with dementia while also staying well?

As a carer, looking after yourself is essential to sustaining a positive, supportive, long-term relationship with a person living with dementia. However, finding the time and energy to stay well can be a challenge. Someone in the early stages of dementia is likely to remain relatively independent, their life not particularly different from how it was before their diagnosis. As the disease progresses, it will increasingly fall to carers to support them to dress, prepare and eat meals, take medication, exercise, socialize, and help with their hygiene.

Some people with dementia increasingly rely on their carer as a point of security. Not being near their carer can intensify anxiety, stress, and distress. Under these conditions, carers can struggle to find time to look after themselves – their own physical and emotional needs, keeping in contact with family and friends, and following their interests.

In many countries, unpaid carers are entitled to financial and practical support. It is no exaggeration to say that, without unpaid carers, national economies would buckle. Recent research carried out by Carers UK estimates that unpaid carers save the UK government £132 billion annually, an average of £19,336 per carer. As such, carers' rights to financial and practical support are enshrined in legislation.

Many family members are reluctant to identify as a carer. They worry that doing so makes them less of a husband or wife, partner, son, daughter, or friend. Contacting your local authority or carers organization should not change the nature of your relationship but is the first step to finding out about the range of available support and potentially striking a healthy balance between caring for a person with dementia and caring for yourself.

How can I manage my emotions?

Carers may experience various, sometimes contradictory, emotions, including denial, anger, resentment, guilt, loss, and even acceptance. It is important to acknowledge these feelings when they arise and remember that they are normal. There is no need to feel ashamed.

Denial

After diagnosis, many carers will convince themselves that the person with dementia is not ill. They put changes in the person's mood, behaviour, and abilities down to ageing. Others will believe that dementia isn't a progressive disease; think that when the person with dementia experiences a 'good' day, they are improving or recovering. As the symptoms of dementia intensify, it can be hard to maintain a state of denial.

Anger, frustration, and resentment

Carers can find it hard to accept that the person with dementia can no longer do what they used to be able to do. As the person becomes more reliant, it is easy to resent the new role and additional responsibilities. These are usually on top of the responsibilities you had before and come at the expense of doing the things you enjoy. It is also easy to resent relatives who don't appear to be pulling their weight to help you and the person with dementia. Carers can often feel abandoned and isolated.

Guilt

Guilt is perhaps the most common emotion we hear carers express. Carers may feel guilty for a variety of reasons:

- for feeling angry or frustrated with the person they care for, especially when they express these emotions
- for resenting the impact caring has on their life: a husband did not envisage spending his retirement caring for his wife; a daughter did not expect to juggle childcare, employment, and a fulfilling social life with looking after her father
- for the negative thoughts that can creep in when tired, worried, and under immense stress – perhaps wishing that they could leave the person with dementia or that the person would go away or even die
- regret over things that didn't happen in the past, and for not having been kinder, more loving, or having made more of time together in the past
- because they think they are falling short of unrealistic expectations, or the 'right way' to care.

It is easy for carers to compare themselves to their peers and conclude that they are 'caring wrong' or not coping as well as others. There is no right or wrong way to care. Each caring relationship is unique, like each person's experience of dementia. Carers will learn and adopt approaches that work for them and the person they care for, and adapt as new challenges arise. Spending time with other carers can be valuable support, but remember that everyone deals with challenges and stress differently. For some carers, the presentation of coping can be an integral part of how they continue caring. For others, talking about the difficulties can be a release and what helps them keep going.

The British paediatrician and psychoanalyst Dr Donald Winnicott spoke about being a 'good enough' mother. 'Good enough' is good enough. This applies equally in our context. A 'good enough' carer relies on their sound instincts and trusts that they know the person they care for best. They are open to new ideas but are neither fixated on professional expertise nor prepared to be measured against any ideal. They will always provide their best care they can within their human limitations.

Sometimes carers feel guilty about not being with the person they care for and worry that needing a break is a mark of failure. If you ever feel this way, take a step back and remember that knowing when to ask for help is actually a strength. A breakdown in your health as a carer is ultimately a breakdown in the caring relationship. As a result, the person with dementia may be admitted to a hospital or moved into long-term care prematurely. Moreover, an often unspoken reality is that many people with dementia can benefit from a break from their carers, enjoying different experiences and interacting with others.

Loss

Carers, like the person with dementia they care for, experience a series of losses as the disease progresses. They gradually lose the relationship they had before the onset of symptoms. This change can be devastating for some carers – particularly spouses and partners – who might have been in a relationship with the person for over 50 years. It is incredibly tough to watch the person you love struggle with things that were once second nature and mourn changes in your relationship.

It is normal to feel sadness and to cry, or to keep your emotions to yourself; to withdraw, or else need to see others more often. You might be inclined one way today and the other tomorrow. You might respond differently to the different losses you and the person with dementia experience over time.

Acceptance

Like any other emotional state, acceptance is not necessarily the final word on the matter. You will still experience a range of different feelings, often without warning. Acceptance might mean that you are learning to live in the present with the person with dementia. You understand your emotions and accept all of them, positive and negative, as normal. You might find meaning and satisfaction in caring for someone you love, helping make their quality of life the best you can. You might have found ways to channel 'negative' emotions through friendship, counselling, exercise, or writing. You might have been able to ask for and accept help from others – for the person with dementia and you.

Caring is not a puzzle to be solved once and for all but a fluid, interpersonal relationship based on observation, listening, understanding, and adapting. It is normal to make 'mistakes' and for best intentions to go wrong. No carer is or can be perfect. Every carer will run out of patience, lose their temper, and occasionally raise their voice in frustration. Try to avoid self-criticism and forgive yourself when this happens. You will not always be able to help how you feel, but you might be able to determine how you respond to your feelings.

How can I cope practically?

Taking positive practical steps can help you come to terms with and adapt to the changes in your life and to cope with your emotions.

Approaching practical tasks

A previously successful approach to supporting the person you care for to take a shower might suddenly stop working. If this happens, take a step back from the situation. Remember that the person you are caring for is not trying to make your life difficult.

They are experiencing gradual but profound changes in their abilities. Evaluate what the new obstacles to taking a shower might be. Are they unsure of how to get into the shower? Are they afraid of the water falling over their head? Do they no longer recall how to wash independently? Or do they feel a loss of dignity because they need support? Try to put yourself in the person's shoes to assess each stage of any task from their perspective. You can then identify and hopefully address the underlying issues causing or contributing to the person struggling with the task or refusing your support.

Establish good routines

Establishing a routine when everyday life feels so unpredictable can be hard. However, a good routine, including a realistic and reliable set of tasks, activities, and timings you can follow, can give you and the person you care for a sense of familiarity and control. Any routine needs to balance other priorities, such as looking after grandchildren, caring for someone other than the person with dementia who is unwell, or going to work (or all three!). Try to work out the things you *really* need to do and those that are less important; do the most pressing first. Likewise, focus on the decisions you can make and those elements of life you can control, accepting those you can't. You are only one person, and it is impossible to do everything.

Establish an informal support network

Many carers benefit from talking about what they are experiencing and how they feel. Sometimes they speak to family and friends. At other times, they don't want to burden these relationships with their perceived 'negativity', or they get the sense that they're not fully understood. Other carers of people with dementia are most likely to know what you are going through. Sharing advice and supporting each other emotionally and practically can significantly reduce feelings of isolation and stress. Many carers form new friendships after meeting in peer support settings, and their conversations extend beyond tips for caring.

It remains sensible to speak with family and friends about how you feel, and guide them on how they can help you and the person you care for. Can someone spare a couple of hours? Not only is this a break for you, but it is another meaningful relationship for the person with dementia. Can someone offer practical help, such as shopping or helping with your financial management? Delegation benefits you and family and friends who might feel unsure what they can do or who have limited time. Recognizing your limits and asking for help when needed will help you manage your emotions, stay physically well, and sustain your caring relationship longer.

Connect with formal supports

Many carers are reluctant to engage with social care services (such as care at home and replacement care) too soon. They worry that to do so is to begin a new stage of life, perhaps prematurely. These concerns are understandable. However, it is helpful to identify and address issues as they arise, adding layers of support gradually instead of waiting for a crisis. If the situation is an emergency, care services will not always be able to respond as sensitively, and professionals can take decisions out of your hands. Making timely contact with dementia and carer charities and community organizations – for information, advice, and peer support – can be a good staging post before requesting formal practical support.

Both dementia and carer charities can be valuable sources of information, advice, and practical and emotional support in their own right. When caring for a person with dementia there might not always be a straightforward solution. However, regularly talking with an experienced, empathetic person can go some way to helping you adapt and cope.

Take a break!

Many carers feel guilty if they are not spending all their time with the person with dementia. They worry that needing a break is a mark of failure. Some carers also doubt the quality of replacement care. Will a family member, friend, or voluntary or paid support be able to provide the quality and consistency of care they do? Perhaps more pertinently, many carers find it difficult to source replacement care from overstretched professional services.

All that said, it is essential to find time to take regular breaks to rest, relax, socialize, follow your interests, or even catch up on outstanding jobs. Time out will not only help you cope better and provide care for longer but can also reduce the person with dementia's dependency on you by showing that they can enjoy other meaningful relationships.

Short breaks at community groups, activities, and day services for people with dementia are available in most areas. Paid one-to-one support or voluntary befriending schemes can also form part of your routine. In some areas, it is also possible to arrange regular overnight breaks. Find out about the financial allowances available where you are. This additional income can help pay for or top up funded care provision. Additional income could also be used to pay cleaners or gardeners, for example. Such support might free up time to enjoy your relative's company or to take time for yourself.

Look after your own health

Caring for a person with dementia can be a full-time occupation and is likely to take its toll on your physical, mental, and emotional wellbeing. Even when you are not with the person with dementia, you will often worry if they are OK and being well looked after. It can be hard to switch off.

Take care of yourself. Try to eat a well-balanced diet, exercise regularly, and maintain a good sleep pattern. Manage pain, and seek treatment as appropriate for any health conditions.

Consider how much you can realistically cope with and what your triggers are. Develop coping mechanisms to help you remain calm and stay as well as possible. Know when and who to ask for help. You might also consider assistive technology to help with the practical elements of care and to monitor your health.

20

Other questions we were asked...

Why do I remember how I felt but not what I did?

Difficulties recalling short-term memory is usually one of the first things people notice when dementia develops. In contrast, emotional memories are often unaffected by the brain changes of dementia or are only affected at a much later stage.

As a result, a person with advanced dementia can still feel what it is like to be with a loved one even if they cannot recognize them. A relative of one of Tom's patients put it well when he said his wife doesn't recognize him anymore, but 'she knows me'.

The endurance of emotional memories is also one of the main reasons you might benefit from continuing to participate in social activities and other positive experiences. You might not always recall what happened for very long afterwards, but the feelings of connection and happiness remain. Positive emotional experiences can help you live well with dementia by improving your mental health and motivating you to stay active. The opposite is also true. Negative emotional experiences linger, can depress your mental health, and affect your future choices. If you felt unwelcome in a group, you might decide against returning. If another person upsets you, you might try to avoid their company. Negative emotional memories can also be barriers to your carer providing support. If you have felt embarrassed or belittled by how your carer has spoken to or treated you, you might be more reluctant to allow them to help. Resolving negative emotional memories can be difficult if you can't always put your feelings into words. Carers might find they are second-guessing what is on your mind, and your perception of what made you feel bad, and their perception could be very different.

Why can I remember what happened a long time ago but not what I had for lunch?

There are various ways to classify different types of memory. One of which is to distinguish long-term memory from short-term memory. We can go further and separate what we call 'working memory' from short-term memory. Working memory is what we used (before mobile phones!) when we looked up a number in the telephone directory, walked across the room to the telephone, and dialled the number. Once the telephone number is no longer needed, you forget it.

However, many things make their way from working memory into short-term memory. But how short is short term? A rough rule of thumb is a matter of hours to days. Memories of this duration are often the sort that someone with dementia struggles with, resulting in them repeating the same stories or questions. Longer-term memories from earlier in life tend to be more robust. For example, many people can remember the names of their primary school friends but not what they had for breakfast.

Why does the person I care for act differently with friends or health professionals?

This perplexing and frustrating phenomenon is experienced by many carers and family members. It is sometimes referred to as 'showtime'.

Carers can be frustrated by this in two ways. First, the person with dementia they care for seems able to 'perform' for other people. Second, this performance can make it more difficult to get necessary support. Communicating separately with the doctor or other professional can help them get a full and accurate picture of the situation.

What is going on here? They are not being manipulative, and their symptoms are not 'put on'. Instead, the person is responding how most people would in a situation where they feel threatened.

Faced with a health or social care professional who the person with dementia might not remember (or may never have met), they might instinctively feel afraid. They do not want to receive bad news. That could be the initial diagnosis of dementia or something else. The person might therefore downplay or not disclose symptoms and challenges and instead try to paint a picture that suggests there are no serious issues.

Furthermore, the person's dignity is at stake. They do not want to share information suggesting their independence and abilities are diminishing. They might understandably consider this embarrassing.

Finally, denial – both as a defence mechanism and to put off receiving bad news – might lead them to refuse to acknowledge and accept the challenges they are experiencing. Some people with dementia are simply unaware of their symptoms.

A 'performance' can't last very long; it requires a lot of effort. Afterwards, carers might find the person exhausted and more confused and agitated. People with dementia typically place the most trust in those carers who they know best. In their company, the full extent of the challenges they are experiencing soon becomes apparent again.

Carers can find this experience not only perplexing and frustrating but isolating. Professionals, other family members, and friends – who often spend only short periods with the person – might not believe the carer's account of their experience. As a result, carers in this situation can feel alone and unsupported.

It is often best to speak openly with family and friends about your experience as a carer and the challenges the person with dementia is experiencing. Not everyone will want to know the reality. This may be because they think it will mean more responsibility or because they want to think of the person as they were without dementia. Nevertheless, they could still help by taking on specific tasks, such as shopping or collecting prescriptions, leaving you more time to focus on providing direct care.

Afterword

This book was not intended to be read from cover to cover, but rather to be dipped into as and when necessary. However, it seems appropriate to try to bring the various questions together here at the end of the book. Each person with dementia is unique, but we hope that everyone will find something useful in these pages. We have enjoyed working together on this book and have found that our experiences – Tom as a doctor working in the NHS and Michael working in a charity which provides care and support to people with dementia – have fitted together well and complemented each other. Like many people living with dementia and their families, one thing we both look forward to is an effective treatment for dementia. As we have mentioned, there are several trials of potential treatments which are due to report soon, so we live in hope.

If something happens which we haven't covered anywhere, we include contact details for several local dementia charities who are likely to be able to help you in your specific situation. We have also mentioned some books, articles, films, and websites which we have enjoyed or found useful.

Further resources

Books

Lisa Genova (2015) *Still Alice*. Simon & Schuster.
Andrea Gillies (2009) *Keeper: A Book about Memory, Identity, Isolation, Wordsworth and Cake...* Short Books.
Oliver James (2009) *Contented Dementia*. Vermillion.
Wendy Mitchell (2019) *Somebody I Used to Know*. Bloomsbury.
Wendy Mitchell (2022) *What I Wish People Knew about Dementia: From Someone Who Knows*. Bloomsbury.

Articles

Alzheimer's Association (2022) Alzheimer's Disease Facts and Figures. Available at: www.alz.org/media/documents/alzheimers-facts-and-figures.pdf
Gill Livingston et al. (2020) Dementia prevention, intervention, and care: 2020 report of the Lancet Commission. *Lancet* **396**: P413–46. Available at: https://doi.org/10.1016/S0140-6736(20)30367-6
Rebecca Mead (2013) The sense of an ending: an Arizona nursing home offers new ways to care for people with dementia. New Yorker 20 May. Available at: www.newyorker.com/magazine/2013/05/20/the-sense-of-an-ending-2
UK Government (2022) Cognitive decline, dementia and air pollution: a report by the Committee on the Medical Effects of Air Pollutants. Available at: www.gov.uk/government/publications/air-pollution-cognitive-decline-and-dementia

Films

Lost for Words (1999, dir. Alan J. W. Bell) with Thora Hird and Pete Postlethwaite (adapted from Deric Longden's autobiography)
Iris (2001, dir. Richard Eyre) with Judi Dench and Jim Broadbent (based on John Bayley's memoir)
Away from Her (2006, dir. Sarah Polley) with Julie Christie and Gordon Pinsent (adapted from Alice Munro's short story)
Still Alice (2014, dir. Richard Glatzer and Wash Westmoreland) with Julianne Moore (adapted from Lisa Genova's novel)

Websites

Alzheimer Disease International
www.alzint.org

Alzheimer's Europe
www.alzheimer-europe.org

Alzheimer Scotland Dementia Research Centre
www.alzscotdrc.ed.ac.uk

Dementia Services Development Centre
www.dementia.stir.ac.uk

Dementias Platform UK
www.dementiasplatform.uk

Join Dementia Research
www.joindementiaresearch.nihr.ac.uk

NRS Neuroprogressive & Dementia Network
www.nrs.org.uk/dementia

Playlist for Life – Personal music for dementia
www.playlistforlife.org.uk

Rare Dementia Support
www.raredementiasupport.org

UK Dementia Research Institute
https://ukdri.ac.uk

World Health Organization
www.who.int/news-room/fact-sheets/detail/dementia

Local dementia charities

Alzheimer Scotland
24-hour Freephone Helpline 0808 808 3000
www.alzscot.org/

Alzheimer's Society (England & Wales)
Direct Connect Support Line 03330 150 3456
www.alzheimers.org.uk/

Alzheimer's Society (Northern Ireland)
National Helpline 0300 222 1122
www.alzheimers.org.uk/

The Alzheimer Society of Ireland
National Helpline 1800 341 341
https://alzheimer.ie/

Alzheimer's Association (USA)
24/7 Helpline 800.272.3900
www.alz.org

Alzheimer Society of Canada
Referral service 1-855-705-4636
https://alzheimer.ca/

Dementia Australia
National Dementia Helpline 1800 100 500
www.dementia.org.au

Alzheimers New Zealand
Dementia support 0800 004 001
https://alzheimers.org.nz/